Madness at the Theatre

Madness at the Theatre

Femi Oyebode

RCPsych Publications

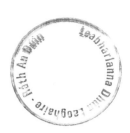

© The Royal College of Psychiatrists 2012

RCPsych Publications is an imprint of the Royal College of Psychiatrists,
17 Belgrave Square, London SW1X 8PG
www.rcpsych.ac.uk

British Library Cataloguing-in-Publication Data.
A catalogue record for this book is available from the British Library.
ISBN 978 1 908020 42 0

Distributed in North America by Publishers Storage and Shipping Company.

The views presented in this book do not necessarily reflect those of the Royal College of
Psychiatrists, and the publishers are not responsible for any error of omission or fact.

The Royal College of Psychiatrists is a charity registered in England and Wales (228636) and in
Scotland (SC038369).

Printed by Bell & Bain Limited, Glasgow, UK.

Contents

Preface

This is a book about the theatre, about dramatic representations of madness, about the emblems and devices that are deployed to signal madness in the theatre. Conduct, bodily posture, gait, gestures and facial expressiveness, language, and dress are some of the ways that are used to communicate madness to the audience. Why is this subject of interest to a psychiatrist? Psychiatry is principally concerned with psychopathology and this is determined by careful observation of conduct, posture, gait, gestures and language among other things. Attention to language, to the explicitly stated, to the overt meaning, the unsaid and covert meaning, the *mis*-said and *mis*-heard, are part of the stock in trade of psychiatry. Dramatic dialogue, particularly since Henrik Ibsen and in Harold Pinter, relies on the ambiguity of language, the very aspects that psychiatrists too work with in the clinic. Therefore, it stands to reason that the crafts of the dramatist, the actor and the psychiatrist have much in common.

To elaborate on these points further, when a psychiatrist sees a patient who is dressed in bright colours, who is restless, jovial and exuberant, he is likely to conclude that a mood disorder is likely to be present. This is the same thing as saying that manifest behaviour is interpreted as a sign of internal, emotional experience. In the theatre, this same principle is at play: the actors signal internal, inner feeling by visible behaviour. In this, at least, there is a correspondence, if inverse, of method and interest between clinical psychiatry and the theatre. Thus, this book is about the symbolic representation of madness in the theatre and it suggests that codes and conventions exist for denoting mental states. How far these conventions borrow from the behaviour of the mentally ill and how far the theatrical codes themselves influence the behaviour of the mentally ill is uncertain but worth pondering. Do the mentally ill, by a process of cultural osmosis, come to know what is 'expected' of them when in a disturbed state? Are psychiatrists too inculcated into these codes both by their training and by cultural osmosis? There are, as yet, no definite answers to these questions. But, it is intriguing to consider the origins of the many and varied behaviours that denote and signal emotional turmoil and psychiatric pathology.

The overarching thesis of this book is that over historical time there is a clearly delineated trajectory of the methods of denoting madness in Western and Western-influenced theatre. This trajectory moves outwards from unobserved but described behaviours in Greek tragedies to fully observed, truly tragic and public enactments of madness on a grand, Shakespearian scale. Following from this grand method, there is the domestication of madness in the theatre, that is, madness is brought within the smaller but more intimate setting of families in the late 19th and early 20th centuries, particularly in the works of Ibsen. Thus, the displays of madness are more readily made a part of daily life, a part of the potential scenarios within the life story of the middle classes. In the 20th century, the importance of the personal history of the writer in the development of both character and plot became obvious. It was not merely that madness had been domesticated, as in the theatre of Ibsen, but also that the springboard for the enacted madness was the dramatist's own life or that of his family. This is taken as proof of the authenticity of the account. This development is best exemplified in the works of the American dramatists Tennessee Williams and Eugene O'Neill. Two further developments take place. One, that personal madness, aberrant and deviant behaviour in the individual, is more a reflection of a society that has gone mad and not merely a sign of personal malady. This view has echoes in the anti-psychiatry movement of 1960s, especially as espoused by R. D. Laing. The idea is that the mad individual is only symptomatic of a mad world, a visible reaction to that world. This is a recurring theme in Wole Soyinka's theatre. Second, the theatrical space is itself a mirror of the internal world of the dramatist. This is in contrast to the idea that the theatre is a mirror of life, of public experience shared with others. Hence, the words spoken on the stage are embodied, but nonetheless, echoes from the inner world of the author. If the author is disturbed, even suffering from psychosis as in the case of Sarah Kane, then these voices are akin to auditory hallucinations, spoken aloud such that the audience can enter into the author's world. There is a sense in which all theatre is a window into the inner world of the dramatist. However, Sarah Kane pushes the limits of this obvious fact. She portrays her own inner world without the usual conventions of characterisation and obvious plot. But, at least the voices are embodied. The next possible stage in the development of theatre, if one were to take forward this line of reasoning, would be simply to have an empty stage with nameless, unidentified and disembodied voices declaiming by virtue of hidden loudspeakers to truly mirror a subjective and abstract mental space.

To summarise, my thesis is that a demonstrable progression of method and system exists in the portrayal of mental illness, of madness in the theatre. This is often invisible and implicit in the dramatic works. Yet, it is there to see and has implications for the perception of madness by the lay public and perhaps also for patients and psychiatrists. The choice of plays and playwrights is not arbitrary but intentional. The plays and dramatists that best illustrate my thesis are emphasised. In developing my thesis about madness in the theatre, I am aware that my argument is itself set in the context of developments in dramatic method in general over the period that I discuss. Greek tragedies were set in the polis, in public and the language and personae were hieratic. Later, more modern works utilised different strategies to deepen the influence on the emotions of the audience. These strategies of demotic language use, of ordinary settings, of surprising and unpredictable shifts of internal logic are distinct from the manner in which madness is itself enacted but there are intersections of purpose, correspondences of conception that are outside the scope of this book.

In this book, I have travelled back in time to the Classical Greek period and forward from then to our own time in the 21st century, always attending to how madness is treated and how that informs the concerns of a psychiatrist. Classical Greek tragedy eschewed public enactment of madness but the spoken accounts were immensely vivid and continue to influence literary descriptions to date. The depiction of Heracles (or, as he was known by the Romans, Hercules) as he fights imaginary opponents is practically indistinguishable from that of Mrs Rochester in *Jane Eyre*. It is thus possible to catch a glimpse of the original model of madness in Western literature. Greco-Roman comedy exhibited comic folly to public view. This was, so to say, the safe face of madness; as it was comic it did not frighten the audience. Folly was easier to play and unaccompanied by dread.

It was Shakespeare who brought tragic madness to the full purview of the public. What before him had been merely described was now enacted in all its horror and dreadfulness. Shakespeare left a rich legacy of delusional jealousy, induced jealousy, melancholia, disintegrative madness, pretended madness, folly and more in his plays. These varied and complex conceptualisations of madness allow for an exploration of the accepted conventions of theatrical madness of his day. For example, pretended madness relies on the codes that actor and audience in collaboration agree signal madness. But, how is this to be distinguished from 'true' madness? What is it that separates malingering from authentic madness given that both are only being acted? There is more too in Shakespeare that is of interest to the psychiatrist. There is, for example, the fact that he instructs his audience as to his method. He teaches them how to interpret facial expressions, what inner emotions and particular behaviours point towards, and so on. This is a master class in descriptive psychopathology.

Where the Greeks and Shakespeare had dealt with princely families, Ibsen brought madness into domestic situations and showed how ordinary people might be afflicted despite their ordinariness. Madness was thus democratised. Heretofore madness had brought the mighty low, had reversed their fortunes. In Ibsen, madness was not a distant affliction but a contemporary event, occurring in families that looked and spoke like the audience. The origins were not far-fetched but close to home and the audience was potentially vulnerable. For all this, Ibsen was often using madness as a metaphor for emotional corruption, a symbol of penance and retribution, and of stigma. In other words, the point was not to accurately capture the nature or origin of madness but to symbolise something else. His interest was not in madness itself but in the nature of family dynamics in a hypocritical society, in how women respond to the oppressiveness of patriarchal society and so on. Nonetheless, Ibsen's characterisation of madness humanised it, made it easier, first, to imagine madness, second, to imagine madness affecting someone that members of the audience knew and loved.

It was Tennessee Williams' treatment of mental illness that focused on the illness itself, not merely as a symbol or metaphor but as a subject in its own right. He fashioned his mad characters from personal and intimate knowledge, drawing faithfully from his sister's history. In Williams, madness was centre stage. However, it was never merely as a study of madness but always exploring and investigating the nature of memory, of insight, of manners and of human relationships even when impaired by illness. This was an updating of Ibsen. The characters were observed within families, hence the power and toxic aspects of family life were scrutinised, much as Ibsen had done. In Williams, however, it was madness itself that was of interest and was portrayed fully and unambiguously, yet with respect.

The next development in this trajectory of the portrayal of madness in theatre was that adopted by Wole Soyinka. He inverted the dramatic mirror to hint that personal madness may be a response, indeed a reasonable response, to the collapse of society. In his drama, the personal is a symbol of collective folly. Both the individuals in the play and the context of the play are deemed mad. The madness of the characters is rendered comprehensible by the social context, the absurdity of war or despotism, for instance. Once again we witness a reversal in the treatment of madness. Here the interest is not in the personal agony of the character, neither is it to do with accuracy of description or understanding of the psychological logic of the progression to disintegration. Rather, madness is a symbol, a metaphor for the ills of society. This is not to say that the characters are not believable or that they are merely ciphers, for they are not. It is to emphasise that the works are not concerned with individual suffering. For a psychiatrist, Soyinka's approach exemplifies what is already a maxim, that context can often render what is opaque and mysterious about a psychiatric case, open to interpretation and understanding.

In the last chapter, I argue that the English dramatist Sarah Kane's later works are the logical culmination of the development of how madness has been treated in the theatre. She wrought of her own mental anguish a theatre of such melancholia and bleakness that it stands as a tribute to all individuals who are afflicted by madness. But, it is less for this reason that she is of interest to a psychiatrist. Her work is, in essence, the display of her internal subjective space on a public platform for the scrutiny of all. The internal subjective space is the abstract space in which mental life is conducted. Psychopathology, by definition, exists in this space as it pulls and distorts the perception and relationship with objective reality that the person experiencing it has. The characters in these later plays, if they can be called characters, are embodied but nameless voices. These characters have all the features of 'voices', auditory and verbal hallucinations that are the hallmarks of psychosis. In these works, the audience is exposed to the apparently structureless, but nonetheless powerfully evocative, disturbing world of the author. The authenticity of the audience's experience of this mad world is guaranteed as the author has manifestly truly had these experiences.

This book is an exploration of Greek tragedy, through Greco-Roman comedy, to Shakespeare, to the modern theatre of Ibsen, Williams, Soyinka and Kane. Madness journeys from invisibility on the Greek stage to full presence, indeed to such exposure in Sarah Kane's work that the audience is immersed totally in the inner world that constitutes madness.

We ought not to need reminding that madness is a serious, tragic sickness. It is not mere poetic metaphor. It is very real. Yet, it is part of the human condition. Like disease and death, it is feared but attracts attention, interest, and stigma. This book shows the manifold ways in which madness is understood and represented. This wider place of madness as a concept within society is, in my view, part of the field of interest of psychiatry.

Femi Oyebode

CHAPTER 1

Greek tragedy and models of madness

Greek tragedy as practised by Sophocles, Aeschylus and Euripides was already a mature art form. The origins are lost but probably included theatrical enactments for religious purposes. The place of masquerades for religious purposes in contemporary African societies is probably as close as one will get to these early developments of theatre in the Western tradition. In these festivals, the masquerade was not merely *representing* the spirit or animal but *was* that spirit or animal. The re-enacted triumph of war, the dramatised recovery from illness or the play of hunter and hunted had not only representational power but also an authentic coalescence of symbol, myth and reality that had cathartic power and authority. The mask and costume transcended the symbolised object and merged with it. So, when the masquerade danced or sang, it was really the represented object dancing or singing. This aspect of theatre, the blurring of illusion and reality to make a magical world that was a transfigured real world was there in the Greek theatre and rendered theatre a more potent force. This feature still remains in our day too, but is significantly, severely diluted. Greek tragedy relied on this potency to accentuate its dramatic action and to evoke its emotional impact.

Aristotle (384–322 BC), in *On the Art of Poetry*, described tragedy as 'a representation of an action that is worth serious attention, complete in itself, and of some amplitude; in language enriched by a variety of artistic devices appropriate to the several parts of the play; presented in the form of action, not narration; *by means of pity and fear bringing about the purgation of such emotions*' (my italics) (Aristotle, 1965 edition, pp. 38–39). This reference to 'pity and fear' and 'the purgation of emotions' signals at once the importance of psychological processes not only to the construction and enactment of tragedy, but also to the inner experience of the audience. For Aristotle, pity is 'awakened by undeserved misfortune' and fear 'for someone like ourselves' who suffers (p. 48). These feelings presuppose in the audience the capacity for empathic engagement with the characters and their situations, a capacity to imagine the world of the characters and experience it in oneself. This is proof of the role of tragedy in depicting, exploring, evoking and commenting on the emotional life of the audience. It was this aspect of tragedy that Freud understood and borrowed from in describing the Oedipus complex. Freud also borrowed from Aristotle's reference to the 'purgation of such emotions' in the audience. The capacity of the plays to impel and sublimate emotions must be understood in the context of the syncretism of symbol and object, and the power of this syncretic world to evoke a space that was immanent with significance, with danger, with urgency, and that was portentous. This is the transfigurative potential of the theatrical space.

In *Oedipus Rex*, an example of complex tragedy, Sophocles (496–406 BC) constructed and exemplified the markers of great tragic drama: individual transgression as the source of social pollution; undeserved reversal of social status; recognition and self-knowledge as determinants of tragic reversal of fortune; and finally, the semiotics of madness in tragedy. In this chapter as in the rest of this book, I will argue that these markers have continuing importance in contemporary society and that they point to aspects of social and intrapsychic life that underlie many of the disquieting circumstances that present to psychiatrists.

This exploration of Greek tragedy is not an attempt at archaeology; there is no intention to dig up what the plays may have meant to a Greek audience 2000 years ago or what the plays tell us about how Greeks understood madness. The force of my argument will be directed at the ever-present relevance of these plays in modern life and in particular to illuminating the recesses of inner life. Underlying this endeavour is an awareness of how texts reveal as much as they conceal, just exactly as words behave in the clinic – as Davies (1992) put it, 'words may hide feelings and intentions better than silences by serving as a smokescreen' (p. 63). Part of the craft of every psychiatrist is to sense what is below the surface dialogue, to apprehend that which is out of reach. Playwrights and psychiatrists alike share this skill of sensitive awareness to the complexity of dialogue. Again, Davies (1992) referred to this similarity between dramatic dialogue and psychiatric interviews when he wrote: 'much is left below the surface, and there is an iceberg of hidden meaning, just as there often is in conversations in the consulting room' (p. 62). There is an additional limitation inherent in language, namely that there are experiences, often emotional experiences, which are recalcitrant to description. In drama this gulf can be remedied by enactment of the imagined experience; here, the bodily replaces the verbal as a means of expression.

Individual transgression and social pollution

Oedipus Rex opens with the Priest saying (quoted from the Grene & Lattimore edn, 1968):

> A blight is on the fruitful plants of the earth,
> A blight is on the cattle in the fields,

a blight is on our women that no children
are born to them; a God that carries fire,
a deadly pestilence, is on our town

(lines 25–29)

The state of affairs described here is the result of individual transgression, the double infamy of unwitting murder of Laertes by his son Oedipus and Oedipus sleeping with his mother Jocasta and having children by her. This causal attribution of social malady to an individual's conduct and the special status of the killing of a blood relative and of mother incest as uniquely transgressive acts is at the centre of the play. What is unusual to the modern mind is the locus of causation. This is not merely the breeching of a taboo, an infraction against a social prohibition regulated by custom and inviting sanction. The adverse material and physical consequences described in *Oedipus Rex* are neither symbolic representations of social pollution, nor allegory for social corruption. Rather, it is that the material and moral worlds are co-extensive, that individual action influences the moral world and the material world simultaneously, that there is intimate correspondence between these worlds.

In our time natural disasters are no longer regarded as resulting from individual social transgression. No one asks why an earthquake or tsunami occurred expecting an answer that draws attention to the murder of a blood relative or mother incest. Disasters in the material world require technical explanations, not appeals to moral understanding of causation. However, this seeking for moral answers continues in vestigial form in clinics. It is still the case that patients ask the question 'Why me?' when diagnosed with an incurable illness, meaning 'What did I do to deserve this?'. The technical answer that explains the biology of the illness misses the point and leaves the patient dissatisfied because a technical answer will not do for a moral question. In psychiatric clinics, in individuals with depression the ideas or delusions of guilt can take the form of the person feeling responsible for adverse events in the natural world, so that personal acts that the individual considers shameful may be thought of as responsible for natural disasters or the deaths of others, sometimes happening thousands of miles away. These are vestiges of the core belief that sustains *Oedipus Rex*, namely that balance in society, the good of society requires adherence to normative values, that there is deep correspondence between individual acts, social order and the material world. Cleansing is accomplished by exile, a true expulsion of the corrupting influence in order to restore, to make reparation for the insult against the body politic.

A number of Greek tragedies have this conceptual framework, at least as a buttress if not the whole foundation. Aeschylus' *The Oresteian Trilogy* deals with the return of Agamemnon from Troy, his murder by his wife Clytemnestra, her murder by her son Orestes, and Orestes' subsequent trial. The murder of Clytemnestra by her son – the killing of a blood relative

– required a sitting of an Athenian court and special pleading by Athena. It is perhaps in *The Oresteian Trilogy* that we get closest to a balancing of arguments to establish the relative merits of the murder of kin in contrast to the murder of others. In *The Choephori*, the second play in the trilogy, Orestes says (quoted here from the 1956 edition, transl. Vellacott):

> It was no sin to kill my mother, who was herself
> Marked with my father's blood, unclean, abhorred by gods,
> And, for the spells that nerved me to this dreadful act,
> I offer, in full warrant, Apollo Loxias,
> Who from his Pythian oracle revealed to me
> That if I did this deed I should be clear of blame;
> If I neglected it – I will not tell the penance.

(lines 1026–1032)

In counter-argument, his mother responded in the third play, *The Euminides* (in Vellacott, 1956):

> I am held guilty and condemned; while, for the blow
> My own son struck, no angry voice protests. See here,
> This wound under my heart, and say whose was the sword!

(lines 100–102)

In *The Euminides*, the Chorus of the Furies, in a long passage, indicts Orestes for the murder of his mother:

> This is his trail, I have it clear. Come, follow, where
> The silent finger of pollution points the way.
> Still by the scent we track him, as hounds track a deer
> Wounded and bleeding. As a shepherd step by step
> Searches a mountain, so we have searched every land,
> Flown wingless over sea, swifter than sailing ships,
> Always pursuing, till we gasp with weariness.
> Now he is here, I know, crouched in some hiding-place.
> The scent of mortal murder laughs in my nostrils –
>
> .   .   .   .
>
> No hope can rescue him.
> A mother's blood once spilt
> None can restore again;
>
> .   .   .   .   .
>
> Mark this: not only you,
> But every mortal soul
> Whose pride has once transgressed
> The law of reverence due
> To parent, god, or guest,
> Shall pay sin's just, inexorable toll.

(lines 244–252, 260–262, 267–272)

Euripides' *Medea* also draws on the same conceptual framework, for when Medea murders her two sons in order to spite Jason, she has to flee Corinth for Athens. The murders of Jason's betrothed and of her two sons are calculated and performed in cold blood. Medea says in preparation (quotes from Vellacott, 1963):

> But in my plot to kill the princess they must help.
> I'll send them to the palace bearing gifts, a dress
> Of soft weave and a coronet of beaten gold,
> If she takes and puts on this finery, both she
> And all who touch her will expire in agony;
> With such a deadly poison I'll anoint my gifts.
> However, enough of that. What makes me cry with pain
> Is the next thing I have to do. I will kill my sons.
> No one shall take my sons from me. When I have made
> Jason's whole house a shambles, I will leave Corinth
> A murderess, flying from my darling children's blood.
> Yes, I can endure guilt, however horrible;
> The laughter of my enemies I will not endure.

(lines 785–797)

When Jason discovers her actions, he wails:

> You abomination! Of all women detested
> By every god, by me, by the whole human race!
> You could endure – a mother! – to lift sword against
> Your own little ones; to leave me childless, my life wrecked.
> After such murder do you outface both Sun and Earth –
> Guilty of gross pollution?

(lines 1325–1330)

What these tragedies trade on is that these murders are especially abhorrent and leave the perpetrator unclean. In *Oedipus Rex* the socially polluting dimension is explored. This reading of *Oedipus Rex* emphasises the adverse power of the breaching of socially prohibited behaviour, even if as we see in the tragedy, the murder and incest are unwitting and not wilful. Freud's interpretation by contrast emphasises elements that are not even by implication in the play: 'The boy's Oedipus complex, in which he desires his mother, and wants to get rid of his father as a rival' (Freud, 1933: p. 166). For Freud, the destiny of King Oedipus 'moves us only because it might have been ours – because the oracle laid the same curse upon us before our birth as upon him. It is the fate of all us, perhaps, to direct our first sexual impulse towards our mother and our first hatred and our most murderous wish against our father' (Freud, 1997). Freud's assertions may be true but they are not exemplified in the Greek tragedy. The pity and fear that Aristotle refers to when examining the nature of tragedy arises from the undeserved reversal in fortune that in Oedipus' case derives from unwitting murder of his father and mother incest. Indeed, *Oedipus Rex* is different from *The Oresteian Trilogy* and *Medea* precisely because the prohibited acts were not wilful but yet resulted in reversal of fortune.

The degree to which the modern reader *cum* audience is distant from this conceptual framework is a measure of how far modern man is atomised and separated, emotionally and ideologically, from society, how disengaged he is from a sense of community as a cohesive and organic entity. But the distance is not as great as we may imagine. Social transgression might not be accorded cosmic significance, but the transgressor is still treated by social exclusion as if he remains polluting and society protects itself, secluding the individual who transgresses the body politic. We see this in the revulsion for child sexual abuse and the social condemnation and treatment of perpetrators, even in prison.

Reversal of fortune

Aristotle had a lot to say about the role of reversal of fortune in tragedy. He made the point that for reversal of fortune to work it must involve undeserved misfortune, because this arouses our pity and fear that it has happened to someone like ourselves. It is also important that this reversal is not from misery to prosperity but the reverse, from prosperity to misery. The reversal ought not to be due to depravity but to error. In tragedy, the reversal of fortune appears to emphasise the inherent instability of human life and puts the audience on notice for the possibility of radical change in their position. This point is not merely expressed in the action of the play but adumbrated at the end of the play. In *Oedipus Rex*, the Chorus says at the very end:

> You that live in my ancestral Thebes, behold this Oedipus, –
> him who knew the famous riddles and was a man most masterful;
> not a citizen who did not look with envy on his lot –
> see him now and see the breakers of misfortune swallow him!
> Look upon the last day always. Count no mortal happy till
> he has passed the final limit of his life secure from pain.

> (lines 1524–1530)

Euripides uses a formula of words at the end of many of his plays that echoes Sophocles' Chorus at the end of *Oedipus Rex* (this quote is from *Medea*):

> Many matters the gods bring to surprising ends.
> The things we thought would happen do not happen;
> The unexpected God makes possible;
> And such is the conclusion of this story.

> (lines 1416–1419)

This emphasis on the nature of endings underlines the often ignored importance of the ending as a source of interest. There is a natural curiosity about where the trajectory of a life might terminate. It is as if any of us can witness only a few life endings and are instinctively curious about how things will turn out, possibly as a model of how to live, a moral compass to journey by. In tragedy the unexpected happens, predictable happy endings are rare and just desserts uncommon, serving to underscore the unpredictability of the course of life.

The character of the reversal of fortune varies, from blindness, exile and destitution in *Oedipus Rex* to death in Aeschylus' *Agamemnon*. In both Euripides' *Electra* and Aeschylus' *The Choephori* Orestes goes mad. Here we have madness as a disvalued state that symbolises a reversal of fortune. In other words, this is a state to provoke both our pity and our fear. This ending does not depend on the representation or depiction of madness for its effect; it traffics on an already established conduit, namely a collective repository of symbolic meaning and value. This accretion of value and feeling is extant in contemporary culture and is responsible for the pity, fear, shame, self-loathing and stigma of madness. But there is more. In tragedy, to quote Meisel, we are immune from the reversal, 'Our position as privileged witness has brought us into intimate contact with ... the worst thing that could possibly happen to a man: to kill one's father and sleep with one's mother, however inadvertently; with what it feels like to make the discovery, and to realize that one has brought it on oneself while trying to evade it. Oedipus has passed from summit of life and fortune to the deepest abyss; and we, however shaken, remain where we sit' (2007: p. 234). It is not always true that we are immune to the trauma. In most cases, as Meisel says, theatre is an opportunity to experience at arms' length the reversal in the fortune of another person and 'remain where we sit'. But, it can also be an occasion to witness the fall from grace of another person from the standpoint of someone in a similar station, to see in the mirror a reflection of one's own abyss, and to feel just that less isolated, taking comfort in Oedipus' situation.

This fascination with the reversal of fortune of others, a pleasure in the misfortune of others, or *Schadenfreude*, has a powerful force in human affairs. It motivates the contemporary preoccupation with the lives of so-called celebrities, particularly with the reversals in their fortunes, their falls from grace. Moral life, it seems, requires cautionary tales and these are served up in great theatre or in the trivia of gossip columns.

Discovery and recognition

In *Oedipus Rex*, discovery and recognition, in particular self-recognition, forms the gusset as well as the bodice of the play. Oedipus from the opening lines is set upon the course of discovering who he is, aided by the various personages who come on stage to reveal aspects of his story. In other tragedies where discovery and recognition feature, even where the plot turns on the nature of the discovered facts and on the recognition of one person by the other, in comparison to *Oedipus Rex*, these devices are hardly ever the very purposive drive of the play. There are discovery and recognition scenes in both Sophocles' and Euripides' versions of *Electra* and in Aeschylus' *The Choephori*. But it is in *Oedipus Rex* that discovery, recognition and reversal are so intertwined – the change from ignorance to knowledge and the revelation of identity lead to the reversal.

The Greek audience would already have known the story of Oedipus, so that the enactment including the commentaries of the Chorus was operating at several levels. When Oedipus proclaims 'who so among you knows the murderer | by whose hand Laius, son of Labdacus, | died – I command him to tell everything' (lines 225–228), the proclamation would have had an ironic tone to the audience, both exacerbating Oedipus' ignorance and accentuating the tragic momentum. He then declares: 'upon the murderer I invoke this curse – | whether he is one man and all unknown, | or one of many – may he wear out his life | in misery to misery doom' (lines 246–249). The dramatic irony in *Oedipus Rex* 'entails the unstated, or even misstated, but understood' (Meisel, 2007: p. 179), somehow implying a subtext that the audience are omniscient like the gods but unable to assist Oedipus, who has to make his own choices exactly as the audience have to in their ordinary day-to-day lives.

In *Oedipus Rex*, blindness, sight, insight and wisdom are played out in verbal exchanges as well as in conduct. Teiresias-the-seer is blind and Oedipus, who wisely solved the riddle of the sphinx and who has sight, is in ignorance of his own real identity. This set of circumstances allows ample room for irony, innuendo, and in the final accounting, exacerbates in the audiences' light Oedipus' lack of knowledge. Teiresias says pointedly:

> Alas, how terrible is wisdom when
> it brings no profit to the man that's wise!
> This I knew well, but had forgotten it,
> else I would not have come here.

(lines 316–319)

In response to Oedipus' taunting regarding his blindness, Teiresias retorts: 'You have your eyes but see not where you are | in sin, nor where you live, nor whom you live with' (lines 414–415).

This interplay of sight and insight focuses on the importance of sight, of the eyes as a symbol of knowledge. Plato, in *The Republic*, uses the simile of the cave as a representation of the ascent of the mind from illusion to pure philosophy, which is a form of vision that distinguishes substance and shadow (Lee, 1955). The irony here is that Oedipus who has sight has no knowledge but Teiresias who is blind is knowledgeable. Max Byrd (1974) has drawn attention to Pope and Swift's continuing use, in the Augustan period, of the symbolism of light and darkness as stand-ins for reason and evil. This tradition continued through to the 20th century and was notably exemplified in Jose Saramago's novel *Blindness*.

In parallel with this subtle exploration of the nature of knowledge, Sophocles also asks the question whether self-knowledge at all costs is fruitful or whether it carries risk. Oedipus' persistent questioning of his origins, the incessant seeking after self-knowledge, leads inexorably to grief. At one point Jocasta cries out, 'God keep you from knowledge of who you are!' (line 1069).

Oedipus Rex is essentially an uncovering of layers of misapprehension to reach down to an inner layer, a truth unknown to the self, but known to others who witness the gradual stepwise self-discovery that is itself the basis of reversal in fortune. As Nietzsche put it, 'Sophocles saw the most suffering character in the Greek stage, the unhappy Oedipus, as the noble man who is predestined for error and misery despite his wisdom, but who finally, through his terrible suffering, exerts a magical and beneficial power that continues to prevail after his death' (1993: p. 46).

In our time, through the influence of psychoanalysis, there is an expected or assumed association between self-knowledge and personal growth, and the latter is valorised – not merely valued but overvalued. What we encounter in *Oedipus Rex* is the tragic consequence of self-knowledge. In this schema self-knowledge is transformative and, again to draw from Meisel, 'inherent in the form of the drama is the possibility, indeed the expectation, of transformation; a transformation of the situation of the personages as we originally find them; a transformation of the state, in the audience no less than in the personages, from ignorance to knowledge, from innocence to experience, from desire to fulfillment and (or loss)' (Meisel, 2007: p. 18). However, the transformation in Oedipus is a fall from grace, a loss of sight, status and country. In the audience, transformation transpires through catharsis, a purification of the soiled space, a casting aside of the polluting subject and symbolically a purgation of fear, the horror and disgust at the effects of transgression. Oedipus' own positive transformation occurs later in *Oedipus at Colonus*.

Madness

In *Oedipus Rex* madness is the explanation for the repulsive action that takes place off-stage, namely Oedipus' blinding of himself. We never see Oedipus perform the act, we only learn from one of the Messengers that when Oedipus saw 'his wife hanging, the twisted rope round her neck', he tore the brooches fastening her robes and dashed them into his own eyeballs. When Oedipus already blinded comes back to the stage, the Chorus says:

> This is a terrible sight for men to see!
> I never found a worse!
> Poor wretch, what madness came upon you!
> What evil spirit leaped upon your life
> to your ill-luck – a leap beyond man's strength!
> Indeed I pity you, but I cannot
> look at you, though there's much I want to ask
> and much to learn and much to see.
> I shudder at the sight of you.

(lines 1298–1306)

We never see what it is like to act under the influence of madness but the message is clear: only madness can explain the extraordinary. The Chorus presses Oedipus for further explanation:

> Doer of dreadful deeds, how did you dare
> so far to do despite to your own eyes?
> what spirit urged you to it?

(lines 1326–1328)

Oedipus responds that it was Apollo that brought 'this bitter bitterness, my sorrows to completion, | But the hand that struck me was none but my own' (lines 1329–1331). This is an interesting response that raises questions about the relationship between mad acts, consciousness, the will and responsibility, questions that remain with us still today.

Madness in drama is problematic for several reasons. At least in the public eye, madness is the obverse of reason, a territory outside the boundary of experience, and it symbolises through speech and action whatever lacks meaning. Yet, literature and drama have to be coherent, driven by an internal logic that must be comprehensible and made reasonable. Oedipus' action is already meaningful given the reversal of fortune, but the act of self-blinding is regarded as dreadful, even repulsive, and has therefore to be explained as only possible under the influence of madness. Oedipus' reply to the Chorus brings Apollo into the picture. This attribution of the motive force for actions to the gods in Greek culture has been discussed by Simon (1978): 'If a man acts irrationally, it is because a god is carrying out a carefully calculated plan to help one hero and hurt another. There is a method to human madness and human folly, but the method belongs to the mind of the gods' (p. 71). But, as we see in Oedipus' response, he takes responsibility for his actions – 'the hand that struck was none other than my own'. The god Apollo and 'madness' appear to be functioning at the same level, as explanations or a form of excuse. Furthermore, madness also seems to have arisen out of unbearable conflict: how is a man to act whose identity is other than he knew it to be and whose unwitting conduct has transgressed deep social prohibitions, in such a way as to retain dignity?

Simon argues in this regard that 'The heroes of tragedy who go mad (they are always *driven* mad) do so when their world is collapsing around them. Their madness is part of a frantic attempt to hold on to what they know and think right' (p. 90).

There are other examples of madness wrought and enacted, but still away from the full gaze of the audience where the description allows us to more vividly imagine what it is to be mad and to act in the grip of madness. In Euripides' *Heracles* madness is personified and he appears before us, describing what he will do to Heracles (quoted from *Euripides: Medea and Other Plays*):

> …as I strike
> Heracles to the heart, shatter his house, rage through
> His rooms, killing his children first; he who is doomed
> To be their murderer shall not know they are the sons
> Of his own body, till my frenzy leaves him. Look!
> See him – head wildly tossing – at the starting-point,
> Silent, his rolling eyeballs full of maniac fire;
> Breathing convulsively, and with a terrible
> Deep bellow, like a bull about to charge, he shrieks.

> (lines 862–870)

Although we do not witness Heracles' mad behaviour directly, we have a good account from the messenger:

> His face had changed; his eyeballs rolled unnaturally,
> Showing their roots all bloodshot; down his curling beard
> A white froth trickled. Then with a maniac laugh he cried
>
> .   .   .   .
>
> Then he pretended he had a chariot; leapt in,
> Gripped on the rail, and, like a man using a goad,
> Kept thrusting. All his servants looked at one another,
> Laughing yet terrified, saying, 'Is this a joke
> Our master's playing on us, or is he raving mad?'
>
> .   .   .   .
>
> Then he unpinned
> His cloak, stood naked, and began a wrestling-match
> With no one; then proclaimed to an invisible crowd
> Himself as victor.

> (lines 931–933, 940–944, 958–961)

Heracles' conduct culminates in the killing of his sons and wife. Eventually, he falls unconscious and then asleep. When he wakes to the devastation that he has caused, he says 'I understand nothing that I should understand' (line 1105), for he has amnesia for his actions. In *Heracles*, we have a semiotics of madness, signs that both the actors and audience can recognise as denoting madness. These include sudden onset of derangement that is not necessarily understandable in context, bodily gestures such as rolling eyeballs, maniacal laughter, pretend actions, violence resulting in uncharacteristic conduct, and recovery.

Even though these signs are still being developed and negotiated between audience and playwright, and not enacted to public gaze, they are recognisable to us today, for example in Charlotte Brontë's description of Mr Rochester's wife in *Jane Eyre*. In this sense madness in drama is symbolic, a motif, but as Feder says, 'something of the nature of madness itself as an incorporation of the very values and prohibitions it challenges' (1980: p. 4) continues to come through in literature. Inscribed into the descriptions of Heracles' mad conduct are the values, the boundaries that they breach: filial piety, the place of play in adult affairs, etc.

Often, a psychiatrist's preoccupation is with accuracy of description, by which is usually meant verisimilitude of the representation. Undoubtedly, the 'madman of literature is to some extent, modeled on the actual one, but his differences from such a model are at least as important as are his resemblances to it: he is rooted in mythical or literary tradition in which distortion is a generally accepted mode of expression; furthermore, the inherent aesthetic order by which his existence is limited also gives his madness intrinsic value and meaning (Feder, 1980: p. 9). But, it is also possible that the 'actual' madman takes his cue from the literary one. To announce one's madness is also to speak in the symbolic language of madness, the symbol that will be recognised for what it means.

In Sophocles' *Ajax* we have a study of madness, the resulting stigma and consequent suicide. Where in *Heracles* the madness results in violent deaths of his sons and wife, in *Ajax* madness leads to the slaughter of sheep and cattle as well as their drovers, but the social effects on Ajax's reputation are no less devastating. Ajax's madness arose in the context of Achilles' armour having been awarded to Odysseus. What ensued can be interpreted as a form of jealous anger. The goddess Athena said that she 'was there to goad and drive [Ajax] deeper into the pit of black delusion' (lines 59–61; quoted from the 1953 edn). In this account we have Ajax taking the beasts for human prisoners, roped up and marched to his tent where bound to a stake they were tortured. We hear from the Chorus how with the telling of Ajax's conduct, 'fun grows' and 'from mouth to mouth the mocking laughter rises' (lines 150–151). The references to the shame attendant on Ajax are expressed variously: 'Tis powerful tale they tell, and its offspring is shame on all of us' (lines 172–173); and, 'the story is loud in the mouths of the people, and grows on their powerful tongues to a mighty clamour. I fear what is coming to us. He is branded with shame and marked for death' (lines 223–228).

When he recovers and discovers his acts, Ajax cries in aguish and sits 'utterly dejected' (line 320). The Chorus chimes:

Ajax, your champion, whom you sent away
So valorous, lies here, a sorry sight,
Brooding alone,
Cribbed with a sickness of the mind
Past human cure.

(lines 612–616)

The Chorus concludes:

It is better that death should take a man diseased
And wandering in the maze
Of madness...

(lines 632–634)

Madness in *Oedipus Rex*, *Heracles* and finally in *Ajax* proceeds from mere explanation of an act that we do not witness (Oedipus' self-blinding), through to acts of gross violence that result in murder. In *Heracles* and *Ajax*, we hear about the visible manifestations of madness, how madness appears to our apprehension, how it renders the man unconscious of his actions and may be accompanied by amnesia, as in Heracles' example. Finally, the stigma of madness is at least part of the reason for Ajax's suicide. In addition, in these plays madness is presented as occurring suddenly and ending equally abruptly. Ajax's madness results from the disappointment that Achilles' armour was given to Odysseus and also because of Athena's displeasure at Ajax's undue pride – Ajax had been dismissive of her assistance. And thus we have the beginnings of a theory of causation.

In Euripides' most complete tragedy, *The Bacchae*, a theory of causation is more fully developed. The plot is superficially simple: Pentheus rejects the Bacchic rites and has Dionysus arrested. Following this, he is persuaded to secretly watch the Bacchic rites whereupon his mother and other women, on discovering he is there, kill him. The underlying thesis is that to resist the lure of wine, to reject the basic and deep urges to dance and connect to primitive instinct will result in death (quoted from the 1973 edn, translated by Vellacott):

...After her came
Dionysus, Semele's son; the blessing he procured
And gave to men is counterpart to that of bread:
The clear juice of the grape. When mortals drink their fill
Of wine, the sufferings of our unhappy race
Are banished, each day's troubles are forgotten in sleep.
There is no other cure for sorrow. Dionysus,
Himself a god, is thus poured out in offering
To the gods, so that through him come blessings on mankind.

(lines 278–286)

Pentheus' rejection of Dionysus is described by Teiresias as follows:

Foolhardy man! You do not know what you have said.
Before, you were unbalanced; now you are insane.

(lines 366–367)

Dionysus renders Pentheus mad. The manifestations of madness are by now a well-established picture:

There I made a mockery of him. He thought he was binding me;
But he neither held nor touched me, save in his deluded mind.
Near the mangers where he meant to tie me up, he found a bull;
And he tied this round the bull's knees and hooves, panting with rage,
Dripping sweat, biting his lips; while I sat quietly by and watched.

(lines 623–627)

Dionysus, the god of wine in *The Bacchae*, is connected with prophecy, with release of the passions by use of wine. Wine cures sorrows, 'and without wine, neither love nor any other pleasure would be left for us' (lines 779–780). So to reject Dionysus is to turn one's back on love and pleasure. In another tragedy, *Hippolytus*, Euripides explored how the abstemious, chaste Hippolytus is destroyed because of his abhorrence of the bed of love and how unrequited and unconsummated sexual desire on the part of Phaedra leads unavoidably to the tragic outcome of the play. In *The Bacchae*, Dionysus uses his gifts to derange Pentheus and in so doing makes him a figure of fun:

Fill him with wild delusions, drive him out of his mind.
While sane, he'll not consent to put woman's clothes;
Once free from the curb of reason, he will put them on.
I long to see Thebes laughing at him, as he walks
In female garb through the streets; to humble him
From the arrogance he showed when first he threatened me.

(lines 851–856)

Madness also assaults Agaue's (Pentheus' mother's) reason and in her distracted state along with the other female Bacchanals, she kills her son, tearing his arms off, stripping his ribs clean and carrying his head triumphant before her.

The madness evident in these tragedies is stereotyped, occurring suddenly and lasting only for the duration of actions that are outside the range of normal behaviour, and is accompanied by recovery and insight, if not memory of the actions themselves. The madness in these tragedies is not that of an alienated individual revolting against the strictures of social norms, it is a madness that makes possible the breaching of social boundaries, as part of a process of reversal, in which madness is itself the undeserved and tragic outcome or is fundamental to self-knowledge and transformation in the drama. We never witness the mad acts; these are revealed to us in language. There is no mad spectacle; the focus is on language and audition, emphasising the primacy of language and speech quite in contrast to modern cinema, for instance, where the visual is everything. It is also significant that we have no subjective account of the experience, only witness accounts of behaviour that rely on observation and inference. Observable signs of madness, semiotics, rather than self-reports of impairment or abnormal experience, determine what madness is. The range of behaviours, at least the form of mad behaviours, in these tragedies is limited: unusual eye movements, maniacal cries, misidentification of beasts for humans (illusions), and false beliefs such as miming a fight in the mistaken belief that one is fighting an adversary (delusion). In *The Choephori* and *The Eumenides* visual and auditory hallucinations are described as The Furies. It is not simply that madness is a symbol or a device in the tragedies, more that there is teleology to the madness and that it serves a purpose in the drama. Actual madness, of course, need have no moral or meaningful causation. It may have a technical cause, such as abnormal neurochemistry, aberrant neuronal circuitry which operates outside of causal meaning, what Jaspers (1913) referred to as 'genetic understanding'.

In *The Bacchae*, there is a communal dimension to the dramatic action – the female-only Bacchanal rite, acting as a group, wreaks the tragic action by killing Pentheus. This is the opposite pole from *Oedipus Rex* whereby individual action brings about social pollution and disease, and the exile of that individual results in restitution. In *The Bacchae*, the community takes restorative action, and it is a violent action meted out by women with a view to defending the importance of Dionysus, the primeval and instinctual, in the ordering of social life. This signifies the inextricable link between individual and social action: the tragedies are enacted in public space, with the Chorus as citizens witnessing and commenting on the action as it progresses, expressing on behalf of the audience thoughts and opinions that reflect the collaboration of the audience in determining what is expected or seemly. Some of the power of the tragedies lies in the augmentation of the audiences' feelings by amplification in the Chorus who mirrors the audience.

Yet, the symbolism of madness, the desire for the madness to *mean* something, for it to speak something that is comprehensible even though the overt language that the mad character utters is confused, even incomprehensible, is still present in our own world. Patients and their relatives seek meaning in madness, much as the dramatists leverage the madness in plays for symbolic effect. Hence, the delusional content of speech is carefully searched for meaning and the noise of formal thought disorder is scanned for a comprehensible signal. But, perhaps more importantly, the transgressive source of the affliction is sought. Parents feel guilt for the illness of their children, continually seeking the moral origins of this terrible affliction. The logic of narrative coherence demands that events in the social world have a morally comprehensible origin. Greek tragedy operates at this level of reasoning, as does all literature.

References

Byrd, M. (1974) *Visits to Bedlam*. University of South Carolina Press.

Davies, D. R. (1992) *Scenes of Madness: A Psychiatrist at the Theatre*. Routledge.

Dorsch, T. S. & Murray, P. (transl. & ed.) (1965) *Aristotle/Horace/Longinnus: Classical Literary Criticism*. Penguin Classics.

Feder, L. (1980) *Madness in Literature*. Princeton University Press.

Freud, S. (1933) *New Introductory Lectures on Psycho-Analysis* (transl. W. J. H. Sprott). Hogarth Press.

Freud, S. (1997) *The Interpretation of Dreams* (transl. A. A. Brill). Wordsworth.

Grene, D. & Lattimore, R. (eds) (1968) *The Complete Greek Tragedies, Volume 1*. The University of Chicago Press.

Jaspers, K. (1913) *General Psychopathology* (transl. J. Hoenig & M. W. Hamilton). Manchester University Press.

Meisel, M. (2007) *How Plays Work*. Oxford University Press.

Nietzsche, F. (1993) *The Birth of Tragedy* (transl. S. Whiteside). Penguin Classics.

Plato (1955) *The Republic* (transl. D. Lee). Penguin Classics.

Raeburn, D. (transl. & ed.) (1953) *Sophocles: Electra and Other Plays (Electra; Ajax; Women of Trachis; Philoctetes)*. Penguin Classics.

Simon, B. (1978) *Mind and Madness in Ancient Greece: The Classical Roots of Modern Psychiatry*. Cornell University Press.

Vellacott, P. (transl.) (1956) *Aeschylus: The Oresteian Trilogy (Agamemnon; The Choephori; The Eumenides)*. Penguin Classics.

Vellacott, P. (transl. & ed.) (1963) *Euripides: Medea and Other Plays (Medea; Hecabe; Electra; Heracles)*. Penguin Classics.

Vellacott, P. (transl.) (1973) *Euripides: The Bacchae and Other Plays*. Penguin Classics.

CHAPTER 2

Greco-Roman comedy and folly

Tragic madness is hidden from view even though the tragedy is itself enacted in a public space, as 'space in Greek drama bespeaks the polis, the city, its public character reinforced in its choruses' (Meisel, 2007: p. 75). This is in contrast to comic madness that is both a spectacle and an auditory phenomenon in that the madness is visible; it is very much an object of spectacle. The dialogue functions both by itself and underlying the spectacle as it does in tragic drama: 'there in the main to *express*, to *impel*, to *reveal* – express thought and feeling; impel (or defer) changes in condition, situation, and relationship; reveal motives, causes, antecedents, the inner truth or logic of events' (Meisel, 2007: p. 161). In addition to all these, comedy through language aims at the comic and inelegant, at what is absurd and foolish, at the grotesque in human relationships. No doubt comedy like all theatre is a locus of social if not political (especially in Aristophanes) interaction, and a space for psychological projections, but less an arena of ideas, except in Aristophanes where the political and the conceptual are never far apart. In comedy, madness is visible, it is risible and ludicrous; it is also non-threatening.

There is no explicit manifesto of what constitutes great comedy as there is what good tragedy ought to be like. Aristophanes (ca. 446–386 BC), an acclaimed comic playwright of ancient Greece, did not specifically say what he thought distinguished comedy from tragedy, although he was clearly interested in what counted as good tragedy. In *The Frogs* (405 BC) he set up a farcical competition between Euripides and Aeschylus. We have Euripides describing what his contribution to tragedy was in comparison to Aeschylus (quotes from Aristophanes are from the 2005 edition):

EURIPIDES Oh! I have not made horses with cocks' heads like you, nor goats with deer's horns, as you may see 'em on Persian tapestries; but, when I received tragedy from your hands, it was quite bloated with enormous, ponderous words, and I began by lightening it of its heavy baggage and treated it with little verses, with subtle arguments, with the sap of white beet and decoctions of philosophical folly, the whole being well filtered together; then I fed it with monologues, mixing in some Cephisophon; but I did not chatter at random nor mix in any ingredients that first came to hand; from the outset I made my subject clear, and told the origin of the piece.

AESCHYLUS   Well, that was better than telling your own.

EURIPIDES   Then, starting with the very first verse, each character played his part; all spoke, both woman and slave and master, young girl and old hag.

AESCHYLUS   And was not such daring deserving of death?

EURIPIDES   No, by Apollo! 'twas to please the people.

DIONYSUS   Oh! leave that alone, do; 'tis not the best side of your case.

EURIPIDES   Furthermore, I taught the spectators the art of speech…

AESCHYLUS   'Tis true indeed! Would that you had burst before you did it!

EURIPIDES   …the use of the straight lines and of the corners of language, the science of thinking, of reading, of understanding, plotting, loving deceit, of suspecting evil, of thinking of everything…

AESCHYLUS   Oh! true, true again!

EURIPIDES   I introduced our private life upon the stage, our common habits; and 'twas bold of me, for everyone was at home with these and could be my critic; I did not burst out into big noisy words to prevent their comprehension; nor did I terrify the audience by showing them Cycni and Memnons on chariots harnessed with steeds and jingling bells.

(pp. 124–125)

And finally Euripides, who is often the butt of Aristophanes' jokes, says:

EURIPIDES   'Tis thus that I taught my audience how to judge, namely, by introducing the art of reasoning and considering into tragedy. Thanks to me, they understand everything, discern all things, conduct their households better and ask themselves, 'What is to be thought of this? Where is that? Who has taken the other thing?'

(p. 125)

In those passages, Aristophanes has Euripides indicate that his new approach to tragedy included the use of ordinary language, the representation of ordinary people and ordinary (common) habits, and the introduction of reasoning into drama, an invention that Nietzsche argues is a precursor of the New Comedy (Nietzsche, 1993). Thus Euripides introduced the ordinary spectator to the stage, or as Nietzsche put it, 'through him, every man pushed his way through the auditorium on to the stage, and the mirror in which only great and bold features had hitherto had expression now showed the painful fidelity that also reflected the blemished lines of nature' (p. 55). In other words, Euripides closed the gap between the hieratic and the demotic in tragedy and in many ways herein lies the similarity not just with the New Comedy of the Greek dramatist Menander but also with Aristophanes' own approach, the use of ordinary rather than high-flown language and the drawing from ordinary life.

Since in comedy madness is dramatised for comic effect, this limits the range of traits attributable to madness. The intention is not to frighten the audience but to entertain them. This is achieved in the main by interpreting madness as folly. Once again Aristophanes is aware of this distinction between madness as enacted, or better still, described in tragedy and folly which is more benign and akin to cleverness. In *The Cloud* (423 BC), Aristophanes treats the fashionable intellectual beliefs of his day with levity and caricatures Socrates. In the play, faced with legal action for non-payment of debts, Strepsiades, an elderly Athenian, enrols his son in a philosophy school so that he might learn the rhetorical skills necessary to defeat their creditors in court. The son thereby learns cynical disrespect for social mores and contempt for authority and he subsequently beats his father up during a domestic argument, in return for which Strepsiades sets the school on fire. In the following exchanges we hear Socrates described as he 'who knows how to measure the jump of a flea', and yet who is clever to the degree that he and his colleagues 'are never shaved' and 'never go to the baths'. The quoted exchange ends with Phidippides concluding that his father 'has lost his wits', ironically, because of his father's belief in the knowledge of the philosophers:

> STREPSIADES Tis Socrates, the Melian, and Chaerephon, who knows how to measure the jump of a flea.
>
> PHIDIPPIDES Have you reached such a pitch of madness that you believe those bilious fellows?
>
> STREPSIADES Use better language, and do not insult men who are clever and full of wisdom, who, to economize, are never shaved, shun the gymnasia and never go to the baths, while you, you only await my death to eat up my wealth. But come, come as quickly as you can to learn in my stead.
>
> PHIDIPPIDES And what good can be learnt of them?
>
> STREPSIADES What good indeed? Why, all human knowledge. Firstly, you will know yourself grossly ignorant. But await me here awhile.
>
> PHIDIPPIDES Alas! what is to be done? My father has lost his wits. Must I have him certificated for lunacy, or must I order his coffin?
>
> (p. 193)

For Aristophanes, folly and wisdom are contiguous if not co-extensive. The mocking of Socrates and of the Sophists allows Aristophanes to build on the intuitive suspicion of abstruse learning that the common man has and to turn it into a kind of farce. In the *Lysistrata* (411 BC) Aristophanes has Lysistrata convince the women of Greece to withhold sexual privileges from their husbands and lovers as a means of forcing the men to negotiate peace during the Peloponnesian War, a strategy, however, that in the end serves to fuel the battle between the sexes. The play allows Aristophanes to further subvert traditional notions of wisdom, folly and madness. The following quoted exchange makes the point very well:

> L Y S I S T R A T A   Well, for my part, I would say no more. But presently I would come to know you had arrived at some fresh decision more *fatally foolish* [my italics] than ever. 'Ah! my dear man,' I would say, *'what madness next!'* [my italics] But he would only look at me askance and say: 'Just weave your web, do; else your cheeks will smart for hours. War is men's business!'
>
> M A G I S T R A T E   Bravo! well said indeed!
>
> L Y S I S T R A T A   How now, wretched man? *Not to let us contend against your follies* [my italics], was bad enough! But presently we heard you asking out loud in the open street: 'Is there never a man left in Athens?' and, 'No, not one, not one,' you were assured in reply. Then, then we made up our minds without more delay to make common cause to save Greece. *Open your ears to our wise counsels* [my italics] and hold your tongues, and we may yet put things on a better footing.

(p. 146)

This ambiguity between folly and reason, a relationship that ought to be antinomic, but yet is not, is the basis of much of Aristophanes' comedies. Erasmus (1469–1536), in *Praise of Folly*, wrote: 'And, let me tell you, fools have another gift which is not to be despised. They're the ones who speak frankly and tell the truth, and what is more praiseworthy than truth?' (in Radice, 1971: p. 118). It is not just that folly may be the cloak that reason chooses to wear, but that truth too lies within this garb.

I will now go on to show how folly can be instantiated in one personality as in Aristophanes' *The Wasps*, be induced as in Plautus's *Amphitryon*, and enacted and examined by a doctor in Plautus' *The Brothers Menaechmus*.

Malady in *The Wasps*

The Wasps was written in 422 BC and was first produced at the Lenaia festival. The focus of the satire is one of Athens' institutions, the law courts. It is of interest to us because the central character, Philocleon, is described as suffering from a complaint, a malady which is not addiction to gambling, drink or sacrifices, but to attending the courts to cast his vote. Philocleon was a juror. Jurors had to be citizens over the age of 30 and a corps of 6000 were enrolled at the beginning of each year, forming a conspicuous presence about town in their short brown cloaks, with wooden staves in their hands.

The work was voluntary but time-consuming and they were paid a small fee, 3 obols per day at the time of *The Wasps*. For many jurors, this was their major source of income and it was virtually an old-age pension. There were no judges to provide juries with legal guidance and there was no legal appeal against a jury's verdict.

At the beginning of the play we learn that:

> This father has a curious complaint; not one of you could hit upon or guess it, if I did not tell you. – Well then, try! I hear Amynias, the son of Pronapus, over there, saying, 'He is addicted to gambling.'
>
> X A N T H I A S   He's wrong! He is imputing his own malady to others.
>
> S O S I A S   No, yet love is indeed the principal part of his disease. Ah! here is Sosias telling Dercylus, 'He loves drinking.'
>
> X A N T H I A S   Not at all! The love of wine is the complaint of good men.
>
> S O S I A S   'Well then,' says Nicostratus of the Scambonian deme, 'he either loves sacrifices or else strangers.'
>
> X A N T H I A S   Ah! great gods! no, he is not fond of strangers, Nicostratus, for he who says 'Philoxenus' means a dirty fellow.

(p. 5)

The basic if implicit argument is that the love of attending the courts to act as a juror is an addiction comparable with addiction to gambling or alcohol. We are told of the effects of not attending which include insomnia, compulsive ritualistic finger movements, distraction, rumination, and persecutory ideas:

> S O S I A S   'Tis mere waste of time, you will not find it out. If you want to know it, keep silence! I will tell you our master's complaint: of all men, it is he who is fondest of the Heliaea. Thus, to be judging is his hobby, and he groans if he is not sitting on the first seat. He does not close an eye at night, and if he dozes off for an instant his mind flies instantly to the clepsydra. He is so accustomed to hold the balloting pebble, that he awakes with his three fingers pinched together as if he were offering incense to the new moon. If he sees scribbled on some doorway, 'How charming is Demos, the son of Pyrilampes!' he will write beneath it, 'How charming is Cemos!' His cock crowed one evening; said he, 'He has had money from the accused to awaken me too late.' As soon as he rises from supper he bawls for his shoes and away he rushes down there before dawn to sleep beforehand, glued fast to the column like an oyster. He is a merciless judge, never failing to draw the convicting line and return home with his nails full of wax like a bumble-bee. Fearing he might run short of pebbles he keeps enough at home to cover a sea-beach, so that he may have the means of recording his sentence. *Such is his madness, and all advice is useless; he only judges the more each day* [my italics].

(p. 5)

Philocleon's addiction is so severe that his son has tried a variety of remedies, all to no avail. The result is that he is now detained at home:

> S O S I A S So we keep him under lock and key, to prevent his going out; for his son is broken-hearted over this mania. At first he tried him with gentleness, wanted to persuade him to wear the cloak no longer to go out no more; unable to convince him, he had him bathed and purified according to the ritual without any greater success, and then handed him over to the Corybantes; but the old man escaped them, and carrying off the kettle-drum, rushed right into the midst of the Heliasts. As Cybelé could do nothing with her rites, his son took him again to Aegina and forcibly made him lie one night in the temple of Asclepius, the God of Healing, but before daylight there he was to be seen at the gate of the tribunal. Since then we let him go out no more, but he escaped us by the drains or by the skylights, so we stuffed up every opening with old rags and made all secure; then he drove short sticks into the wall and sprang from rung to rung like a magpie. Now we have stretched nets all round the court and we keep watch and ward.

(p. 5)

This malady is not one that we recognise today but as it mimics the addictions to gambling and alcohol we have a good sense of the manifestations. The successful treatment is unusual. Philocleon's house is turned into a courtroom and a case is soon brought before him – a dispute between the household dogs. One dog accuses the other dog of stealing a Sicilian cheese and not sharing it. Witnesses for the defence include a bowl, a pestle, a cheese-grater, a brazier and a pot. As these are unable to speak, Bdelycleon, Philocleon's son says a few words for them on behalf of the accused and then some puppies (the children of the accused) are ushered in to soften the heart of the old juror with their plaintive cries. Philocleon is not softened but his son easily fools him into putting his vote into the urn for acquittal. The old juror is deeply shocked by the outcome of the trial as he is used to convictions. The comedy turns on Philocleon's willingness to act as juror no matter how ridiculous the case and the absurdity is multiplied several times by the troop of witnesses in the shape of a bowl, a pestle, a cheese-grater, a brazier and a pot! There is also irony working at another level: Asclepius, the God of Healing, had failed in this case, yet behavioural manipulation succeeded. But, the cure is not unvarnished; Philocleon's addiction is replaced by addiction to drink, dance, and merriment. This, of course, raises the question of which is preferable, addiction to the courts or to pleasure.

The Wasps publicly portrays madness, even if it manifests as benign foolishness, and the visible manifestations of this madness are subtle: Philocleon's actions are behaviourally unexceptional; he is acting as a juror, but the case he is judging is between two dogs and the witnesses are household utensils. In other words, it is the context of behaviour that determines whether or not it is evidence of madness. This version of madness is different from Ajax killing sheep, believing them to be his human opponents, but at the same time not being fully aware of his actions. Theatre is created as a joint enterprise between the director and audience, where the script 'may be understood as a programme for creating and managing … expectations, and for managing sympathy, antipathy, curiosity, credulity, prurience, revulsion, shock, and deferred gratification' (Meisel, 2007: p. 97). There is a transaction between author, director, actors and audience that is rooted in expectation, the precursor of engagement. Philocleon's madness only works as theatre because there is latent in the audience a notion of what constitutes madness, how madness makes itself manifest, and how far it is liable to respond to treatment and to recovery.

There is also the didactic in theatre. Neely (2004) has argued that:

> '… by representing both madness and the process of reading madness, plays teach audiences how to identify and respond to [madness]. On stage and off, madness is diagnosed by observers – first laypersons and then in some cases specialists. The period's audiences participate with onstage watchers in distinguishing madness from sanity and from its look-alikes: loss of grace, bewitchment, possession or fraud. Madness is represented as a state of dislocation – separated in part from the self who performs and the spectators who watch – but not as a supernatural invasion. For theatre to reach its audiences, it must be readable. For this the stage develops a new form of speech, peculiar to the mad, and cues for how to read it.'

(p. 49)

We are from the outset informed in *The Wasps* that Philocleon has a complaint. The comic madness as dramatised in *The Wasps* can be said to naturalise madness, to domesticate it, render it safe. Philocleon is detained at home, rendered powerless and judging trivial 'cases'. This is not a picture of the feared insane but of a comic, harmless character. This prepares the ground for Samuel Richardson's comments on the pastime of visiting Bedlam: 'I was much at a loss to account for the behaviour of the plurality of people, who were looking at these melancholy objects. Instead of the concern I think unavoidable at such a sight, a sort of mirth appeared on their countenances' (quoted in Byrd, 1974: p. 89).

The double and the induction of madness

In both tragic drama and comedy, either by way of description or enactment, the external signs of madness are often emphasised to the disadvantage of the process or the dynamics of madness, the inner experience of the process of becoming mad. It is obvious why this is often the case; the exterior signs can be 'aped and acted out' (Thiher, 1999: p. 81). This aping and acting out refers only to the exteriority of the experience of madness, and may be incommensurate with genuine expression of inner feelings. Theatre can be conceived of as the external representation of the inner world of the audience wherein 'the inner world of the audience walks on the stage, speaking in lines which articulate unspoken and often unacknowledged feelings' (Oyebode & Pourgourides, 1995). This is not merely a matter of personifying the different elemental aspects of the inner world in order to sharpen conflict and tension, but also a demonstration of how events in the external world can create distance, detachment, alienation and even confusion in the inner world.

Plautus (254–184 BC) was a Roman playwright of the Old Latin period. Plautus' comedies were adapted from Greek models for Roman tastes. *Amphitryon* is described as a tragicomedy. It relies for its comic effect on the concept of the double. The play begins with a prologue by the god Mercury in which he gives some background information to the audience. Amphitryon and his slave Sosia have been away at war and are returning to Thebes. Meanwhile, the god Jupiter is sleeping with Amphitryon's wife Alcmena. Jupiter is in the guise of Amphitryon so that Alcmena is unaware that he is not her husband. Mercury's job is to buy his father Jupiter some time by deceiving those who would interfere. He changes his appearance to look like the slave Sosia, and when the real Sosia arrives, beats him up and sends him away from the house. Thoroughly confused by having been beaten up by himself, Sosia returns to his ship to relay what happened to his master Amphitryon. The following morning, Amphitryon sets off for the house, annoyed by his slave's foolish story. Jupiter leaves only moments before Amphitryon arrives, and when Alcmena sees her real husband, is confused as to why he has returned. Amphitryon does not appreciate this strange welcome after being gone for so many months, and confusion turns to anger and jealousy after learning that she has slept with a man who is not him. After a long argument, Alcmena is ready to leave her untrusting husband but is stopped by Jupiter. He soon begins to set things right, and in a miraculous event, Alcmena gives birth to twin boys. One is the son of Amphitryon; the other is Hercules, the son of Jupiter. To quell Amphitryon's anger, Jupiter explains to him what he did, and Amphitryon is then honoured to have shared his wife with a god.

This is a complex plot. It is a well-known story and both Euripides and Sophocles are known to have composed works based upon it. The use of the concept of the double allows a number of comic effects to transpire but it is the inner subjective experience that is engendered by being confronted by a double of oneself as well as confronting the double of others that is of particular interest to psychiatrists. To understand the nature of these phenomena it is perhaps best to think of what it is like to see oneself in the mirror: the mirror image is, of course, identical and stares back such that the experiencing self feels detached, disconnected, and dislocated from the image. This primal experience signals the nature of alienation from the self, being both oneself and yet not inhabiting that self; this is what the depersonalisation experience is. In addition, the world of the image appears identical but the experiencing self cannot cross the borders of the mirror into the image, therefore the mirror world lacks affective, emotional tone that gives texture to our experience of the world; this is what derealisation is. The primordial nature of this experience is properly realised when the subject of experience suddenly and unexpectedly comes upon himself before a full-length mirror. That initial surprise, that perplexity and instability in the frame of reference is the process–experience that makes the concept of the double so powerful and instrumental in theatre and in literature.

It is this subjective experience that Plautus harnesses and exploits in *Amphitryon* (quoted from the 1995 edn, edited by Slavitt & Bovie):

> MERCURY   I'm Sosia, even though you thought you were.
>
> .   .   .   .
>
> SOSIA   Then listen, I can speak quite plainly now: I am Amphitryon's Sosia.
>
> .   .   .   .
>
> MERCURY   You can't make me be anyone but Sosia.
>
> SOSIA   You can't make me belong to another master;
>
> I'm the only Sosia he has, so help,
>
> The only one he took along to the war.
>
> MERCURY   *The man is out of his mind* [my italics].
>
> (Act I, lines 392, 400, 405–409)

In the end Sosia has to agree that he is not Sosia and he asks 'But look: if I'm not Sosia, who am I?' (line 455) and to himself, panic mounting, he says:

> SOSIA   God help me, now that I look, he has my features –
> I've seen them in a mirror. We could be twins.
> My hat, my clothes – he's more like me than I am:
> Leg, foot, height, haircut, eyes, nose, even lips –
> Jaws, chin, beard, neck – no difference. I'm speechless.
> If his back is scarred he couldn't be more me.
> And yet I'm still the man I was:
> I know my master and my house; *I'm sane* [my italics].
>
> (lines 458–466)

These exchanges and Sosia's subjective response to his situation have relevance to clinical practice because of the phenomena of delusional misidentification syndromes. In 1923, Capgras and Reboul-Lachaud described 'L'illusion des Sosies', a condition that is now termed Capgras syndrome. The essence of this condition is the belief that a person closely related to the patient has been replaced by a double, this despite the fact that the supposed double has physical resemblance to the familiar person. Capgras syndrome is part of a range of phenomena including Fregoli syndrome, the delusion of subjective doubles, the syndrome of intermetamorphosis and reduplicative paramnesia. All these phenomena have at their core an intrinsic belief in doubles as a concept. In Fregoli syndrome, the patient believes that an unfamiliar person who shares no physical characteristics with a familiar person is indeed this person and the delusion of subjective doubles is the belief that a copy of the self who has not been seen is about in the wider world, usually with malevolent intent, perhaps to damage the patient's reputation. Finally, reduplicative paramnesia is the belief that the patient is in an identical place but not the true place; in essence, this is a duplication of place.

Sosia and Alcmena both experience the double; in Sosia's case, this is the double of himself, whereas in Alcmena's case it is the double of her husband. The play is an enactment of the process of how an individual's ground shifts, producing insecurity and at least a questioning of the frame of reference of reality, if not a loss of trust in the parameters of experience.

An experience that would otherwise be alarming and terrifying is in the hand of Plautus amusing and comic. It is as if the toxic and pernicious aspects of madness can be neutralised by comic treatment. Once again, what we see is that comedy inoculates the audience against the possibility of madness as a virulent, violent and horrifying spectacle.

Feigned madness and the doctor

Aristotle (384–342 BC) thought that:

> 'comedy represents the worse types of men; worse, however, not that it embraces any and every kind of badness, but in the sense that the ridiculous is a species of ugliness or badness. For the ridiculous consists in some form of error or ugliness that is not painful or injurious; the comic mask, for example, is distorted and ugly, *but causes no pain*' [my italics].
>
> (in Dorsch & Murray, 1965: p. 37)

There is an emphasis here on comedy causing no pain; in fact, the depictions of ugliness, awkwardness and madness allow for revelry and laughter. Aristophanes in *The Wasps* treats a mental malady with levity, whereas Plautus in *Amphitryon* allows the audience to glimpse the inner confusion that is the precursor of madness in a context that renders it comic and safe. In these comedies and others, there is an avoidance of the kind of madness that we hear about but never see in the tragedies, madness that is threatening and dangerous, that tends towards violence and that results in death of self or others.

In *The Brothers Menaechmus*, Plautus returns to the theme of doubles to create confusion and comic scenes. It is the prototype of Shakespeare's *The Comedy of Errors*. The drama depends on a pair of twins separated from early life and then, unbeknownst to them, reunited during the play. The interest for our purpose lies in the fact that in the play, Sosicles (also called Menaechmus) pretends to be mad and his enactment of madness takes on the manifest garb of dangerous, maniacal madness. In other words, in a comedy tragic forms of madness are only permissible if the audience knows that it is pretend madness, that the actor/character is feigning it (quoted from the 1965 edn, translated by Wattling):

W I F E [*in alarm*]   Look at him, father! His eyes are turning green; all his face is turning green; and that glitter in his eyes – look!

S O S I C L E S [*aside*]   If they are going to declare me insane, the best thing I can do is to pretend to be insane; perhaps that will frighten them off. [*He acts accordingly.*]

W I F E   Now he's gaping and flinging himself about. Oh father, what ever shall I do?

F A T H E R   Come away, my dear, come away as far as possible from him.

S O S I C L E S [*raving*]   Euhoe! Euhoe! Bacchus ahoy! Wilt thou have me go hunt in the woods away? I hear thee, I hear thee, but here I must stay. I am watched by a witch, a wild female bitch, on my left, and behind her a smelly old goat, a lying old dotard whose lies have brought many an innocent creature to ruin…

F A T H E R   Ay, ruin on you!

S O S I C L E S   Now the word of Apollo commands me to burn out her eyes with firebrands blazing…

(lines 826–842)

Here we have the beginning of a semiotics of madness as bodily disposition, inner experience, and use of language: the actor throws himself about, flinging his limbs, with his mouth gaping open; he raves, presumably talking rapidly and responding to a private dialogue that is not heard by the audience, signalling a private, inner and abnormal experience.

How madness is understood and depicted in literature and in theatre in particular is a continuing source of interest. No doubt the Greco-Roman audiences knew what madness was, as no doubt did Renaissance audiences and modern audiences do, and we see something of the convention and public symbols of madness in *The Brothers Menaechmus*. Salkeld (1993), writing about madness and drama in the time of Shakespeare, understood these issues:

> 'It is reasonable to suppose that Renaissance audiences knew the social codes and conventions of how a mad person might look and behave, and would be able to recognise lunacy when they saw it. What then did they see? Clearly not madness *itself*. What they saw was a particular ensemble of symbols which represented madness; a code, historically specific and politically resonant, that signalled unreason. The site of this semiotic code was the body, the space or text wherein the madness was inscribed and represented.'

(p. 3)

In *The Brothers Menaechmus*, the business of determining features of madness is explicitly dealt with. A doctor (psychiatrist) is brought on to the stage to determine whether Sosicles is mad or not (quoted from the 1965 Penguin Classics edn):

> DOCTOR   Now, sir, what did you say was the nature of the illness? Is it a case of possession or hallucination? Are there any symptoms of lethargy or hydropsical condition?
>
> FATHER   I've brought you here to tell me that, and to cure him.
>
> DOCTOR   There'll be no difficulty about that; we'll cure him all right, I can promise you.

(lines 889–894)

There then ensues a number of questions from the doctor: do you drink white wine or red; do you ever feel your eyes scaling over; have you noticed any rumbling in the bowels; do you sleep all night, do you fall asleep easily when you get into bed? As for treatment, the doctor says: 'I'll put you on hellebore for three weeks', and asks that the patient be brought to his house. The doctor adds, 'judging by [Menaechmus'] present condition of insanity' (line 950) not less than four men will be needed to bring Menaechmus to his house.

Menaechmus is surprised to have been pronounced insane and he makes a case for his sanity:

> Exit doctor. Exit father-in-law. Now I am alone. Jupiter! Whatever can have possessed those two to pronounce me insane? Me – who have never had a day's illness in my life! I'm not insane at all, nor am I looking for a fight or quarrel with anybody. I'm just as sane as every other sane man I see; I know my friends when I see them, I talk to them normally. Then why are they trying to make out that I am insane – unless it's they who are insane?

(lines 959–965)

What Plautus makes plain in *The Brothers Menaechmus* is that the semiotics of madness is negotiable. In order to feign madness, the actor has to borrow something from what the audience recognises madness to be. The doctor's role is as much to do with providing ironic tension, diagnosing madness where none exists and thereby undermining the standing of professional expertise, as it is with providing some insight into the technical definition of madness. And, the technical diverges from the public view to introduce themes about possession *v.* hallucination, impairment of vision, abnormal perception of bowel activity, and characteristic disturbance of sleep. Finally, the supposedly insane character argues against the doctor's diagnosis by referring to his physical well-being, his ability to recognise and identify his friends and to have normal speech. This is a complex exploration of competing ideas of madness, even though this play is not about the nature of madness.

Shosana Feldman (2003), in *Writing and Madness*, commented:

> 'Society has built the walls of mental institutions to keep apart the inside and the outside of a culture, to separate between reason and unreason and to keep apart the other against whose apartness society asserts its saneness and redefines itself as sane. But every literary text [which attempts] ... to communicate with madness – with what has been excluded, decreed abnormal, unacceptable, or senseless – by dramatizing a dynamically renewed, revitalized relationship between sense and nonsense, between reason and unreason, between readable and unreadable.'
>
> (p. 5)

Feldman is correct that there is a continuing exploration, dialogue if you wish, between the varying interested parties in defining what madness is. Folk understanding, technical descriptions, and the resistance of the individual to being labelled all jostle for dominant position. Feldman also argues that 'Language discreetly dictates to its users – in an invisible manner – self-evident assumptions and proscriptions that are inscribed in its grammar (which is, by definition, imperceptible from inside the language)' (2003: p. 19).

What is the nature of these assumptions? When Menaechmus says, 'I'm just as sane as every other sane man I see' (line 963), he is also saying to the audience that madness can be recognised by sight. When he says, 'I know my friends when I see them', he is also saying that the insane do not recognise their friends when they see them. The language carries more information than it overtly states. And this speech by Menaechmus demonstrates capacity for reason and underlines the assumption that insanity, unreason and reason are polar opposites. Once again, Feldman is correct when she argues that:

> 'Thoughts, by definition, are the accomplishment of reason, an exercise of sovereignty of a subject capable of truth. I think, therefore I am not mad, therefore I am. The being of philosophy is thenceforth located in non-madness, whereas madness is relegated to the status of non-being.'
>
> (p. 39)

Greek tragedy dealt with the most feared aspects of insanity, imagined danger and violence, and responded to this dimension of madness by rendering it hidden from sight but present in language, hence amplifying the dread in the audience: what is unseen is feared even more for its awfulness. Greco-Roman comedy on the other hand brought folly centre stage, treating malady with levity and making what is commonly fearful the object of laughter and jokes. But this was done in a manner that emasculated the mad, traducing if you wish the mad character to an object of ridicule. This was not a treatment that dignified or made madness comprehensible. In fact, there was little exploration of psychological origins or of the inner world of the mad. The comedies were entertaining at the expense of the mad.

Where the tragedies had hidden madness from view and the comedies had dramatised the absurdities of madness, Shakespeare's approach was to show madness, in its tragic and comical garbs, plainly for all to see. The stage is now set ready for the enactment of tragic madness in full public view in Shakespeare's plays.

References

Byrd, M. (1974) *Visits to Bedlam*. University of South Carolina Press.

Dorsch, T. S. & Murray, P. (transl. & ed.) (1965) *Aristotle/Horace/Longinnus: Classical Literary Criticism*. Penguin Classics.

Feldman, S. (2003) *Writing and Madness*. Stanford University Press.

Ingram, J. & Berger, T. (ed.) (2005) *Aristophanes: The Eleven Comedies, Volume 1*. Project Gutenberg Ebook.

Meisel, M. (2007) *How Plays Work*. Oxford University Press.

Neely, C. T. (2004) *Distracted Subjects*. Cornell University Press.

Nietzsche, F. (1993) *The Birth of Tragedy* (transl. S. Whiteside). Penguin Classics.

Oyebode, F. & Pourgourides, C. (1995) Classical Greek tragedy and the inner world. *Psychiatric Bulletin*, **19**, 362–363.

Radice, B. (transl.) (1971) *Erasmus: Praise of Folly*. Penguin Classics.

Slavitt, D. R. & Bovie, P. (eds) (1995) *Plautus: The Comedies, Volume 1 (Amphitryon; Miles Gloriosus; Captivi; Casina; Curculio)*. The Johns Hopkins University Press.

Salkeld, D. (1993) *Madness and Drama in the Age of Shakespeare*. Manchester University Press.

Thiher, A. (1999) *Revels in Madness: Insanity in Medicine and Literature*. The University of Michigan Press.

Wattling, E. F. (transl.) (1965) *Plautus: The Pot of Gold and Other Plays*. Penguin Classics.

CHAPTER 3

Jealousy the green-eyed monster and madness in Shakespeare

Greek tragedy had hidden mad behaviour from view but the dramatic and violent consequences, even though not held up as spectacle, remained a powerful and compelling antithesis of the good. In contradistinction, comic madness in Greco-Roman comedy was treated with levity, rendered innocuous and enacted to full public gaze. Plautus in *The Brothers Menaechmus* had begun the process of demystifying the signs of madness by placing side-by-side professional and lay views. This process was fully explored and exploited by Shakespeare in varying degrees in *Othello*, *Hamlet* and *King Lear*.

It is obvious, as Meisel says, that:

> 'Theatre is physical, its means material, belonging to the order of bodies, objects, things. When a play dramatizes inner states, inner conflicts, it does so through corporeal means, principally speech and behaviour of actors, and the cues for doing so are what we find in the script... the skills to read each other's latent thought and feeling are what we, the potential audience, practise everyday of our lives in the everyday world.'

(2007: p. 33)

Meisel goes on:

> 'Reading gesture is critical when it takes on more than illustrative and expressive function, when it conveys meanings beyond the dialogue, which it can qualify or condense into something that feels definitive, like the kiss that seals the union of lovers in stage and film.'

(2007: p. 53)

The problem for the playwright is how to signal madness, a rare condition that is neither seen nor interpreted daily by the audience. In Shakespeare, the action, the body and the language carry the weight of this task. In this chapter, I will examine Shakespeare's treatment of madness in *Othello*, *The Winter's Tale*, *Hamlet* and *King Lear*. These four plays reveal different aspects of madness: the induction of madness by manipulation of the social world;

inexplicable madness that distorts reality; factitious madness that serves the protagonist's purpose and by implication inaugurates for the audience the symbols that denote madness; folly and its relationship to madness; and the tragedy of the disintegration of mental life.

Green-eyed monster

In *Othello*, Shakespeare explores the nature of jealousy, the boundaries of understandable jealousy and its violent consequences. This treatment of jealousy differs from that in *The Winter's Tale*, where it is inexplicable and has not arisen by trickery or understandable antecedents. Jealousy is a complex emotion. By this we mean that unlike fear, sadness, joy and anger, jealousy is a composite of different emotions in response to a situation. This conceptualisation is akin to the idea of primary colours and secondary colours; the former irreducible to other elements and the latter a blend of the primary. Early 20th-century French psychiatrists, including Théodule-Armand Ribot, developed perhaps the most sophisticated notions of jealousy as one of the passions. It is an understanding of jealousy as a mixture of emotions accompanied by affront to self-esteem, the yearning for total possession of the loved object, intense self-doubt, and self-torment (Shepherd, 1961). A modern exposition by White & Mullen (1989) defines romantic jealousy as 'a complex of thoughts, emotions, and actions that follows loss or threat to self-esteem and/or the existence or quality of the romantic relationship. The perceived loss or threat is generated by the perception of a real or potential romantic attraction between one's partner and a (perhaps imaginary) rival' (p. 9).

In the psychoanalytic tradition, jealousy is contrasted with envy. Envy in this schema is an emotion that arises within a dyad – between two people – and relates to the emotions evoked in one party by possessions or characteristics of the other party. It is thought to arise from the mother–infant dyad and is prefaced by the infant's recognition of a distinction between itself and mother. The infant comes to recognise its reliance on mother and envies her the possession (of breasts) that makes it possible for her to satisfy the infant's needs but also makes it possible for those needs not to be satisfied. Jealousy on the other hand is an emotion that arises within a triadic/triangular relationship and relates to the emotions evoked in one party by the relationship between the other two parties. This understanding of jealousy underpins the nature of sexual/romantic jealousy: it is the feeling evoked by the real or imagined relationship between a significant other and another person. Jealousy is thought to have its origins in the so-called Oedipal situation, whereby the child's feelings are aroused by the child's recognition of the parental relationship that by definition excludes the child. Thus, in Freudian terms, this is the primal triangular relationship that sets the template for our experience of jealousy.

Clinical descriptions of jealousy focus on the mistaken belief of the partner's infidelity, incorporating the individual's efforts to furnish evidence of proof of these beliefs, usually supported by an accumulation of trivial incidents and experiences that the jealous person invests with a special meaning (Shepherd, 1961). These descriptions vary from the obviously false (delusional) belief and the understandable but morbid readiness to react in a jealous but unfounded manner to reasonable evidence of infidelity.

Shakespeare's triumph in *Othello* was to demonstrate how an individual can be persuaded of the infidelity of a partner and how under the influence of this mistaken belief he comes to act violently, killing the loved one. Iago says of Othello (all quotes from *Othello* are from *The New Cambridge Shakespeare* edition, 2003):

> The Moor is of a free and open nature,
> That thinks men honest that but seem to be so,
> And will as tenderly be led by the nose
> As asses are.

(I. iii. 365)

The point Iago makes here is that a particular kind of disposition is more liable to be misled, and not only misled but put

> into a jealousy so strong that judgment cannot cure
> …making [Othello] egregiously an ass
> And practising upon his peace and quiet
> Even to madness.

(II. i. 267)

Shakespeare with subtlety instructs the audience how to read in the visage, the gestures and manner of the character's inner feelings and emotions. Othello says to Iago:

> And didst contract and purse thy brow together,
> As if thou then hadst shut up in their brain
> Some horrible conceit. If thou dost love me,
> Show me thy thought.

(III. iii. 93)

In another scene Desdemona says to Othello:

> Alas, why gnaw you so your nether lip?
> Some bloody passion shakes your very frame:
> These are portents; but yet I hope, I hope
> They do not point on me.

(V. ii. 49)

This is drama that requires attentive study of the characters' actions, not merely of what they say, as a pointer to inner life. In this context, these same actions can be misconstrued as denoting a particular state of affairs. Here is an exercise in attesting to the fragility of the relationship between sign and meaning. If words are ready tools for deceiving and manipulating the beliefs of others as Iago successfully demonstrates in relation to Othello, behaviour too can be misread:

> IAGO   As [Cassio] shall smile, Othello shall go mad;
> And his unbookish jealousy must construe
> Poor Cassio's smiles, gestures, and light behaviours
> Quite in the wrong.

(IV. i. 93)

But, it is not simply that behaviour can be misread but that with jealousy, the individual actively seeks behavioural evidence for confirmation of their prior, and predominantly erroneous, beliefs. And here we see how prior expectations imbue neutral events with emotional tone, bias the interpretation of incidental and sometimes random events with significance.

In *Othello*, Shakespeare interrogates the differing ways in which signs and symbols may or may not be faithful to their meanings. This examination includes the use of language as well as the meaning of gestures and bodily expressions, and encompasses the faithfulness of character. In *Othello*, it is not only the fidelity of Desdemona that is at stake but also the very idea of fidelity itself. How reliable are words and gestures in denoting, in the commerce of daily life? Are signs fragile or stable and immutable? What can we trust in such a world? This borderland is inhabited by psychoses. In schizophrenia, for example, commonplace symbols like traffic lights assume unique, idiosyncratic meaning. Neutral stimuli, mundane objects acquire significance. In 'delusional perception', an ordinary object acquires special delusional significance, for example a red pen suddenly comes to signify the imminence of the end of the world as we know it. This anomalous belief is built on the same cognitive system that is uniquely human: the capacity to imbue neutral signs with value and significance. That is the basis of language itself. *Othello* trades in this territory.

Jealousy with its admixture of intense and vacillating doubt, assault on self-esteem, self-torment, sadness and anger is more grist to the mill for a playwright as it allows these multivaried emotions to be explored, displayed and perhaps even exorcised. In the voice of Iago, Shakespeare refers to jealousy:

> It is the green-eyed monster which doth mock
> The meat it feeds on. That cuckold lives in bliss

Who certain of his fate loves not his wronger;
But O, what damnèd minutes tells he o'er
Who dotes, yet doubts, suspects, yet fondly loves?

(III. iii. 188)

Later on Iago says:

Trifles light as air
Are to the jealous confirmations strong
As proofs of holy writ...

(III. iii. 330)

And, Emilia responds to Desdemona's 'I never gave him cause', saying:

But jealous souls will not be answered so.
They are not ever jealous for the cause,
But jealous for they're jealous. 'Tis a monster
Begot upon itself, born on itself.'

(III. iv. 148)

Othello's jealousy is induced by Iago but this jealousy required a rich and ready ground to flourish. In other words, Othello was peculiarly vulnerable to this distraction. He was an outsider, a Moor, liable to take people at face value and there is a hint that he suffered from epilepsy or some other malady. Iago says of him:

My lord is fallen into an epilepsy.
This is his second fit; he had one yesterday.

(IV. i. 46)

Once worked on by Iago, Othello's passions did the rest of the work; jealousy no longer needed external inducement to advance its tentacles into Othello. Tragically, jealousy progressed to madness. The implicit notion in *Othello* is that jealousy in its extreme variant can be indistinguishable from madness. The nature of this madness is such 'that judgment cannot cure' (II. i. 267). Othello 'foams at mouth and by and by | Breaks out to savage madness' (IV. i. 46), and as Desdemona says: 'And yet I fear you, for you're fatal then | When your eyes roll so' (V. ii. 49).

The origins of this madness are evident; it is induced by Iago's malicious handicraft, made possible by Othello's character and social status and aggravated by the natural inner dynamic and progression of the jealous state. Othello recovers his insight at the end and says

Then must you speak
Of one that loved not wisely, but too well;

Of one not easily jealous but, being wrought,
Perplexed in the extreme [my italics].

(V. ii. 346)

Thus, the jealousy in *Othello* is understandable. It is rendered comprehensible by Iago's actions. We can see the origins and trace the arc of development of the erroneous belief and the accompanying passion. In contrast, in *The Winter's Tale*, the jealousy is sudden and irreducible. The consequences are no less violent and vicious but there is no attempt to understand Leontes' malady; it is read as unfounded, false and contrary to the understanding of everyone else in his court. It is also held with undue conviction; Camillo says of Leontes' jealousy (*The Winter's Tale* quotes are from *The Oxford Shakespeare* 1996 edition):

Swear his thoughts over
By each particular star in heaven, and
By all their influences; you may as well
Forbid the sea for to obey the moon
As or by oath remove or counsel shake
The fabric of his folly, whose foundation
Is piled upon his faith, and will continue
The standing of his body.

(I. ii. 116–117)

This description is what constitutes delusional jealousy. In other words, whereas Leontes can be described as suffering from delusional jealousy, Othello's jealousy was induced and rooted in socially comprehensible circumstances. The anxiety and distress of jealousy is apparent in Leontes as in Othello. Leontes says:

Dost think I am so muddy, so unsettled,
To appoint myself in this vexation? Sully
The purity and whiteness of my sheets –
Which to preserve is sleep, which being spotted
Is goads, thorns, nettles, tails of wisps –

(I. ii. 112)

But the centrality of sexual exclusivity and the fear of uncertain and ambiguous paternity to jealousy is more marked in *The Winter's Tale* than it is in *Othello*. Where in *Othello* there is one passage referring to sexual exclusivity –

I had rather be a toad
And live upon the vapour of a dungeon
Than keep a corner in the thing I love
For other's uses ...

(III. iii. 284)

in *The Winter's Tale* Leontes makes numerous references, for example:

There have been,
Or I am much deceived, cuckolds ere now,
And many a man there is, even at this present,
Now, while I speak this, holds his wife, by th'arm,
That little thinks she has been sluiced in's absence,
And his pond fished by his next neighbour, by
Sir Smile, his neighbour – nay, there's comfort in't
Whiles other men have gates, and those gates opened,
As mine, against their will.

(I. ii. 105–106)

This fear of the loss of sexual exclusivity is coupled with a preoccupation about paternity. Leontes, referring to Mamillius, his son, says 'hast smutched thy nose? They say it is a copy out of mine' (I. ii. 101); and 'they say we are almost as like as eggs' (I. ii. 101). When Paulina brings his recently delivered son he exclaims:

My child? Away with't! Even though, thou hast
A heart so tender o'er it, take it hence
And see it instantly consumed with fire.

(II. iii. 138)

This preoccupation has deep biological roots that we share with other species. Sociobiological and evolutionary theory argues that male jealousy probably evolved to minimise sexual betrayal and to assure that the children a man supports are his own (Freedman, 1979). In reptiles, birds and mammals where insemination is the mode of fertilisation, the male cannot always be sure that his own sperm has fertilised his mate's eggs. To the degree that the male invests in the care of the offspring, it is genetically advantageous to make sure that he has exclusive access to the female's unfertilised eggs. There are different strategies to achieve this aim. Male-dominance polygamy as occurs in gorillas is a method of avoiding sperm competition. In some birds the time lag between courting, bonding and copulation is in effect a quarantine period for the detection of alien sperm. The most dramatic and interesting strategies occur post-copulation. These include male mice whose odour is enough to cause a pregnant female to abort and so be ready for re-insemination; and nomadic male langurs who normally kill all the infants of a troop after they drive off the resident males and the usurpers, then quickly inseminate the females. The threat posed by sperm displacement which occurs in insects has produced a series of ingenious countermeasures, such as mating plugs in butterflies, or the ceratopogonid female fly eating the male after copulation but leaving his genitalia still attached. In others, the male may transmit substances that reduce the receptivity of the female, which

37

is postulated to occur in the Aedes mosquito. Some flies use prolonged copulation lasting up to 1 hour or more, in spite of the fact that all the sperm has been transferred during the first 15 minutes of copulation. These strategies all emphasise the importance which animals place in ensuring that the progeny, which they will expend parental investment in, are the result of their own gametes. This sets the scene for a possible explanation of sexual jealousy in our own species and makes more comprehensible, if there was any need for this, Leontes' preoccupation with sexual exclusivity and paternity and his violent response to the birth of the child of whose paternity he was unsure.

Where *Othello* was an interrogation of fidelity in all its aspects, *The Winter's Tale* demonstrated the imperviousness of delusional jealousy to reason or counterargument, the destructive power of jealousy on intimate relationships, and the annexation of physical and murderous aggression by jealous passion to tragic ends.

Factitious madness in *Hamlet*

Much has been written already about Hamlet's mental state (Bynum & Neve, 1985). There has been much dispute about whether Hamlet was melancholic, maniacal, neurotic, neurasthenic, hysterical or a malingerer. The analysis and understanding of Hamlet's character has also been influenced by the predominant theory of human personality of the relevant period – in the 20th century this was psychoanalytic theory. What is clear is that Hamlet is a complex, dark and opaque enough character to generate potentially inexhaustible description and categorisation. That itself is a triumph of the genius of Shakespeare.

There are at least three aspects of Hamlet of interest to a student of human emotions: his grief, his being love-struck, and his madness. These aspects are obviously intertwined but need not be regarded as other than co-extensive. In examining *Othello*, we established the degree to which Shakespeare explored the relationship between expressive gestures and their internal meaning. This included the fidelity of the external sign to the corresponding inner emotion and, in effect, Desdemona's fidelity was itself standing in as a representation of the nature of fidelity itself.

In *Hamlet*, dress code is added to the list of potential signs denoting inner life and we shall we see later in *King Lear* that nakedness and the state of dishabille too have symbolic significance pointing inwards. In *Hamlet*, the colour black signals both mourning and melancholia, the melancholia of Burton's *The Anatomy of Melancholy* (Jackson, 1932), a condition recognised as a disabling pathology. Gertrude says to Hamlet (quoted from *The Oxford Shakespeare Hamlet*, 1987 edition) 'cast thy nightly colour off' (I. ii. 68), to which Hamlet retorts:

… 'Tis not alone my inky cloak, good mother,
Nor customary suits of solemn black,
Nor windy suspiration of forced breath,
No, nor the fruitful river in the eye,
Nor the dejected haviour of the visage,
With all forms, moods, shows of grief,
That can denote me truly. These indeed seem,
For they are actions that a man might play;
But I have that within which passeth show –
These but the trappings and the suits of woe.

(I. ii. 77–86)

Again in this passage we see the fragility of the relationship between sign and its object; the one can be 'played' but the latter which is within is real and 'passeth show'.

But, it is not merely colour of dress that can act as a sign. In a later passage Ophelia says:

My Lord, as I was sewing in my chamber,
Lord Hamlet, with his doublet all unbraced,
No hat upon his head, his stockings fouled,
Ungartered, and down-gyvèd to his ankle,
Pale as his shirt, his knees knocking each other,
And with a look so piteous in purport
As if he had been loosèd out of hell
To speak of horrors, he comes before me.

(II. i. 78–85)

Her father Polonius responds 'mad for thy love?' (II. i. 86). Here we see how Hamlet's state of dress, his pallor come to stand for his purported inner turmoil, which Polonius tentatively interprets as a sign of 'the very ecstasy of love' (II. i. 103), where in this context 'ecstasy' translates as madness.

As Meisel (2007) has argued,

'When dress surfaces in a text, in conversation or preliminary description, it has more to do than cover nakedness. Costume can be enlisted both to conceal and to reveal: to conceal, by characters forwarding their private ends; to reveal, by the playwright adding layers of signification.'

(p. 60)

Later, in *King Lear*, we shall see how dress serves both as a disguise and as an emblem. For the present, it suffices to say that dress code by convention or by suggestion can stand in relation to inner life as expressive gestures do and hence can come to create a tone, an atmosphere, casting a subtle hue on the proceedings so that the audience come to a realisation about the inner world of the character under question. This artifice that playwrights deploy is itself reliant on a natural inclination to make judgements about character and personality, about trustworthiness, reliability and so on, on the basis of appearance and dress. Psychiatrists too use this convention as part of their method for making judgements about inner life, for example, interpreting a colourful dress as evidence of elation or euphoria, thereby signalling mania.

What is the nature of the melancholia that Hamlet suffers? The 'inky cloak' is the external sign of the inner experience that Hamlet describes as follows:

> I have of late – but wherefore I know not – lost all my mirth, forgone all custom of exercise; and it goes so heavily with my disposition that this goodly frame, the earth seems a sterile promontory. This most excellent canopy, the air, look you, this brave o'erhanging firmament, this majestical roof fretted with golden fire – why, it appears no other thing to me than a foul and pestilent congregation of vapours. What a piece of work is a man, how noble in reason, how infinite in faculty, in moving how express and admirable, in action how like an angel, in apprehension how like a god – the beauty of the world, the paragon of animals! And yet, to me, what is this quintessence of dust? Man delight not me – no, nor woman either, though by your smiling you seem to say so.
>
> (II. ii. 291–308)

Here then is Hamlet's description of anhedonia, the inability to experience any joy, indeed to draw any emotion from experiences that would normally cause delight. Hamlet appears to be saying that the origin of this feeling is unknown to him, suggesting that it is not grief that is the precursor. In this description, melancholia is not merely sorrow but an inability to experience joy or pleasure, an unresponsiveness to all that is awe inspiring in the world. Vacillation and indecision are both recognised as part of the symptomatology of melancholia. Hamlet's famous speech 'To be, or not to be – that is the question' (III. i. 57) exemplifies this state of mind. When confidence and self-esteem are undermined by melancholia, this invariably adversely influences decision-making, rendering the individual insecure in their judgements, perilously paralysed by self-doubt, and foreseeing only the potentially disastrous outcome.

In literature, melancholia, like madness, cannot be without an understandable cause. There must be meaningful, readily understandable psychological origin. This urge to seek meaning and explanation is in contrast to the clinical situation where despite such a search no readily identifiable social or psychological causation may be found, where an absence of explicit social origins is accepted as wholly possible and plausible. Polonius, Claudius and others subject Hamlet's behaviour to theoretical exploration. The potential explanations are grief or love. These possible explanations tell us something about the theories of madness extant in Shakespeare's day. Quoting Burton, the sorrow of grief is:

'a cruel torture of the soul, a most inexplicable grief, poisoned worm, consuming body and soul and gnawing the very heart, a perpetual executioner, continual night, profound darkness, a whirlwind, a tempest, an ague not appearing, heating worse than fire, and a battle that hath no end. It crucifies worse than any tyrant; no torture, no strappado, no bodily punishment is like unto it.'

(Jackson, 1932: p. 259)

Grief 'dries up the bones…makes them hollow-eyed, pale, and lean, furrow-faced, to have dead looks, wrinkled brows, rivelled cheeks, dry bodies, and quite perverts their temperature that are misaffected with it' (pp. 259–260).

Finally, love, too, if it tyrannises over men, 'is no more love, but burning lust, a disease, frenzy, madness, hell' (Jackson, 1932: p. 49).

What is clear from these quotations is that in the 16th century, when Burton's work appeared, there were already well-developed explanatory hypotheses that the audience understood and they would have needed little prompting to apply this folk knowledge to Hamlet's case. The descriptions in Burton's *The Anatomy of Melancholy* include bodily experiences, inner experience and expressive bodily gestures. As ever in the theatre, the expressive gestures allow for reverse engineering: bodily habitus, facial and gestural language pointing inwards to emotional life. This point is well made by Claudius:

> …Something have you heard
> Of Hamlet's transformation – so I call it,
> Since not th'exterior nor the inward man
> Resembles that it was. What it should be,
> More than his father's death, that thus had put him
> So much from th'understanding of himself
> I cannot deem of.

(II. ii. 4–10)

Hamlet's madness is confirmed by Polonius:

> I will be brief. Your noble son is mad.
> Mad call I it, for, to define madness,
> What is't but to be nothing but mad?

(II. ii. 92–94)

In Polonius' opinion, the reason for Hamlet's distemper is love for Ophelia.

Much has been written about Hamlet's madness, particularly about whether he was insane or merely feigned insanity (see Bynum & Neve, 1985 for a full discussion). The characteristics of Hamlet's distraction are interesting whether or not he was feigning madness. In his interaction with Polonius in Act 2 Scene 2 his responses to some questions posed by Polonius suggest that he understood them, yet gave the wrong answer:

POLONIUS Do you know me, my lord?

HAMLET Excellent, excellent well. You're a fishmonger.

POLONIUS Not I, my lord.

(II. ii. 173–175)

This is an example of 'talking past the point' or *Vorbeireden*, which is typically described as indicating that the person understands the question but is deliberately talking about an associated topic. Clinical examples include a patient who is asked 'What is the colour of grass?' and who responds 'white'. *Vorbeireden* is said to indicate either deliberate malingering or unconscious motivation for some advantage and was first described by Sigbert Ganser in criminals awaiting trial.

In response to a question about what he is reading, Hamlet produces this monologue:

Slanders, sir; for the satirical rogue says here that
old men have grey beards, that their faces are wrinkled,
their eyes purging deep amber or plum-tree gum, and
that they have plentiful lack of wit, together with most
weak hams – all which, sir, though I most powerfully
and potently believe, yet I hold it not honesty to have it
thus set down; for you yourself, sir, should be as old as I am
– if, like a crab, you could go backward.

(II. ii. 196–203)

It is this speech that prompts Polonius' famous response: 'Though this be madness, yet there's method in't' (II. ii. 104). And further:

… How pregnant
sometimes his replies are! A happiness that often madness
hits on, which reason and sanity could not prosperously
be delivered of…

(II. ii. 207–210)

There is here an allusion to the possibility of meaning in madness, more precisely in mad speech. Even more than that, there is a possibility that mad speech has a special relationship to truth and that the seeming obliqueness or opacity is merely a mask for deeper meaning. This suggests that mad speech has the potential of revealing profundity not to be found in ordinary speech. Surface dialogue may harbour hidden depths just as conversations in the consulting room often do, because words conceal as well as reveal and the revelations may point obliquely rather than directly. This tendency may be more manifest in mad speech than it is in ordinary speech.

There is a paradox here. Mad speech almost by definition is meaningless if not incomprehensible. But literature and drama require words to be meaningful. Therefore, mad speech in drama has to hint at incomprehensibility while at the same time appearing to communicate. Hence the contention by many critics that madness in literature and drama serves to interrogate the boundaries of meaning, that mad speech serves to subvert the social and/or political order of the day. Shoshana Feldman (2003) argues that:

> 'every literary text … continues to communicate with madness – with what has been excluded, decreed abnormal, unacceptable, or senseless – dramatizing a dynamically renewed, revitalised relation between sense and nonsense, between reason and unreason, between readable and unreadable.'
>
> (p. 5)

In *Hamlet*, language and speech become tools for signalling madness. Dress, gesture, facial expression and behaviour have all been deployed in conveying to the audience the idea of madness. To this is now added language. Language as a marker of madness is further developed in *King Lear*. But in *Hamlet*, it is a song (delivered by Ophelia), a variant of speech which is also shown to be a sign of madness. This relationship between language and madness (whether language as song or speech), that is language as a marker of origin and difference, is an intriguing aspect of mad speech in drama. The language of the mad, even though it is the same language that the audience speaks, has to be somewhat differentiated that is it needs markers of difference to indicate the strangeness of madness. Feldman claims (2003) this in itself allows the mad to speak freely as the internal moorings of language can be and are subverted in mad speech. This view that mad speech is free of some of the limitations of ordinary speech is perhaps what Polonius refers to as a 'method in madness'. Ophelia's speech is at once nothing but 'yet the unshaped use of it doth move the hearers to collection' (IV. v. 5–6). And the thought that is had of her botched words is constructed from the hearer's own conjecture as to its meaning. Here we see that communication can work through the listener reconfiguring and rendering meaningful what is said, even when what is said is apparently empty of meaning.

Lilian Feder extends this argument when she writes:

> 'the madman of literature is, to some extent, modelled on the actual one, but his differences from such a model are at least as important as are his resemblances to it: he is rooted in a mythical or literary tradition in which distortion is a generally accepted mode of expression; furthermore, the

inherent aesthetic order by which his existence is limited also gives his madness intrinsic value and meaning.'

(1980: p. 9)

How far extant models of madness influenced the characterisation of Hamlet is impossible to estimate. In addition, whether Hamlet the theatrical character informed folk understanding of madness and then by extension influenced the presentation of actual madness is also impossible to tell. It is likely that these were mutually reinforcing systems. Real madness served as a model for literary or dramatic representation and these literary creations themselves affected how madness was perceived, and may have in turn contributed to the presentation of madness. This is to say that actual madness (the behaviours labelled as mad) took its cues partly from what was expected of a mad person and by this mutually reinforcing process, what psychiatrists see in the clinic and how dramatists and actors represent madness are intimately related.

Hamlet hallucinates his father's ghost, bending 'his eye on vacancy' (III. iv. 110), his 'bedded hair like life in excrements | Start up and stand on end' (III. iv. 115–116). These are all signs of his distraction. He acts strangely, as someone full of apprehension, suspicious of the world, 'mad as the sea and wind when both contend' (IV. i. 6). These added to all the other signs confirm him well and truly mad. In the end, Hamlet excuses himself: 'What I have done ... I here proclaim was madness' (V. ii. 176–178). He continues:

> Was't Hamlet wronged Laertes? Never Hamlet.
> If Hamlet from himself be ta'en away,
> And when he's not himself does wrong Laertes,
> Then Hamlet does it not, Hamlet does it not, Hamlet denies it.
> Who does it then? His madness, If't be so,
> Hamlet is of the faction that is wronged;
> His madness is poor Hamlet's enemy.

(V. ii. 179–185)

We have here a complex argument about the relationship between moral agency and madness, about the structure of the self in madness, and about identity in madness. These matters continue to concern us in today's world.

Disintegrative madness

There are three kinds of madness portrayed in *King Lear*: the truly mad king, the feigned madness of Edgar in the role of Poor Tom, and finally the Fool. Both Lear and Edgar rely on their bodies to dramatise their malady, whereas Tom and the Fool use language to display madness as well as to escape the limitations of unreason. These methods of depicting and playing madness were based upon extant social codes and conventions of how a mad person might look and behave. The Renaissance public well knew lunacy when they saw it and the naked body in a public place was one of its manifestations as it remains today.

Salkeld (1993) argues that the body has a special place in how madness is portrayed:

> 'The body was openly displayed as the object of political, juridical and medical knowledge: a site of power represented in the body of the king, and a site of spectacular violence, of torture and execution in the body of deviant "subjects".'

(p. 56)

He goes on:

> 'Madness is conceived as a disordering or disruption of the normative meaning of the body, signifying a disorder within both subject and state since the head and the monarch share the same rule according to the metaphor of the body politic. Madness is a sign of sovereignty – whether of monarchy or reason – in crisis. Visually, it is displayed on the surface of the body, in its disguises, its disarray and its nakedness, as conventional meanings are thrown into contradiction... Corporeal and sartorial display *enounces* a semiotics of power and identity: the body is staged as a king, father, lover, and seeks recognition within the play's symbolic order. Madness is effected in the contradiction of these hierarchical and conventional orders of meaning.'

(Salkeld, 1993: p. 60)

It is true that in *King Lear*, both the king and Edgar in their madness derive some of the power of their roles from their nudity. Nudity is elemental; it is a recall of the primordial state, of the shedding of dignity, of a return to the most basic manner of living. And as Salkeld suggests, it evinces chaos, a crisis of governance, or the irruption of unreason.

The 'Storm' scene has the king exposed to the ferocity of the elements and this itself was a metaphor for the storm raging abroad and within Lear (*King Lear* quotes are from *The Oxford Shakespeare King Lear*, 2000 edition):

> This tempest in my mind
> Doth from my senses take all feeling else
> Save what beats there: filial ingratitude.

(xi. 12–14)

The exposure to the storm itself symbolised the vulnerability of the naked human body, defenceless and unprotected. Lear and Poor Tom's nakedness gain their meaning and significance from being 'houseless heads and unfed sides' and the more vulnerable for having only Poor Tom's blanket between three people. Lear accentuates the significance of Poor

Tom's nudity when he proclaims: 'Unaccommodated man is no more but such a poor, bare, forked animal as thou art' (I. xi. 95–97) before starting to strip down to nothing himself. Indeed, being a naked monarch who has lost his estate and is unclothed in a storm is evidence of being stripped of civility.

This scene conjoins Lear's nakedness in a storm with the idea of elemental forces at large, forces that render man insignificant, exposed and vulnerable. Furthermore, the outer storm stands in for inner storm of unconscious life. As Feder (1980) put it, 'Shakespeare creates a new prototype: the mad king who naked confronts his own unconscious impulses and motives and forces within nature and society that have determined both his power and his impotence' (p. 119).

When Cordelia later sees Lear, he is:

> As mad as the racked sea, singing aloud,
> Crowned with rank fumitory and furrow-weeds,
> With burdocks, hemlock, nettles, cuckoo-flowers
> Darnel, and all the idle weeds that grow
> In our sustaining corn …

(xviii. 2–6)

Lear's decline was total but restitution was still possible. His disintegration was unusually temporary. Whatever kind of madness it was that the king suffered from, it was not one wherein his wits were permanently lost. Was Lear's madness therefore merely allegorical? Poor Tom's madness was feigned in contrast to Lear's. But, the easy restitution of Lear's faculties suggests that even his madness may not have been the real thing!

The storm scene more than invests the naked body with spectacular power, it also emphasises the way in which mad speech, both as folly and unreason, can go to the heart of truth. The Fool makes apposite comments, Poor Tom moralises, and Lear makes profound statements. But, it is easy only to focus on Poor Tom's strange speeches, such as 'This is the foul fiend Flibberttigibbet' (xi. 103) and 'The Prince of Darkness is a gentleman; Modo he's called, and Mahu' (xi. 129–130) or on his self-description as 'Poor Tom, that eats the swimming frog, the toad, the tadpole, the water-newt and the water; etc' (xi. 115–116).

It is accepted that Shakespeare relied on Samuel Harsnett's book *A Declaration of Egregious Popish Impostures* (1603) for Poor Tom's mad language. Our interest though is that madness in *King Lear* accretes to the characters by virtue of their nakedness and their speech. The madness of Lear, Edgar/Poor Tom and the Fool is centre stage in the storm scene and succeeds as a coherent and comprehensible scene notwithstanding the mad speeches, the ravings, if you wish, of Poor Tom and the inner anguish, psychical tempest and inner chaos of Lear. This is itself what distinguishes theatrical madness and true madness. The one is willed and in aid of a plot, and has narrative drive. The other is motiveless and often unspeakable even when it has speech at its disposal. What unites Shakespearian tragedy and the Greeks is that the drama is about princely families, and the setting and language are elevated, hieratic if you wish. Ibsen's significant contribution was to inalterably change this. His plays were domestic in scale and the language was as ordinary as everyday speech. Ibsen was holding a mirror to the audience such that they saw a reflection of themselves in terms of the stage set, what the characters wore and how they spoke, and their social status and roles. The portrayal of madness in this new theatre was therefore that more full of danger for the audience, as the mad could easily be a neighbour, a relative or oneself.

References

Bynum, W. F. & Neve, M. (1985) Hamlet on the couch. In *The Anatomy of Madness, Volume 1* (eds W. F. Bynum, R. Porter & M. Shepherd): pp. 289–304. Tavistock Publications.

Feder, L. (1980) *Madness in Literature*. Princeton University Press.

Feldman, S. (2003) *Writing and Madness*. Stanford University Press.

Freedman, D. G. (1979) *Human Sociobiology: A Holistic Approach*. Free Press.

Hibbard, G. R. (ed.) (1987) *The Oxford Shakespeare Hamlet*. Oxford University Press.

Jackson, H. (ed.) (1932) *Robert Burton: The Anatomy of Melancholy*. New York Review Books.

Meisel, M. (2007) *How Plays Work*. Oxford University Press.

Orgel, S. (ed.) (1996) *The Oxford Shakespeare The Winter's Tale*. Oxford University Press.

Salkeld, D. (1993) *Madness and Drama in the Age of Shakespeare*. Manchester University Press.

Sanders, N. (ed.) (2003) *Othello. The New Cambridge Shakespeare*. Cambridge University Press.

Shepherd, M. (1961) Morbid jealousy: some clinical and social aspects of a psychiatric symptom. *Journal of Mental Science*, **107**, 687–704.

Wells, S. (ed.) (2000) *The Oxford Shakespeare King Lear*. Oxford University Press.

White, G. L. & Mullen, P. E. (1989) *Jealousy: Theory, Research, and Clinical Strategies*. Guilford Press.

CHAPTER 4

Ibsen and the domestication of madness

Michael Meyer (1967), Ibsen's biographer, has commented that Ibsen made three significant contributions to the theatre. First, demonstrating that high tragedy could be written about ordinary people; second, doing away with well-worn artificial plot devices of mistaken identities, overheard conversations, intercepted letters, etc.; and finally, creating modern male and female characters of depth and complex interiority. High tragedy before Ibsen had taken place in palaces or castles rather than in parlours and sitting rooms. Ibsen showed that high tragedy could be written about ordinary people and in ordinary prose. In so far as Ibsen eschewed hackneyed devices, he developed the art of:

> 'prose dialogue to a degree of refinement which has never been surpassed; not merely the ways people talk, and the different language they use under differing circumstances, but that double-density language which is his legacy, the sub-text, the meaning behind the meaning.'

> (Meyer, 1967: p. 862)

By the exclusive use of this language he propelled the plot forward, revealing or concealing as necessary the motive force of the play. This use of language required a different kind of acting, a departure from the declamatory, recitative mode to a more sensitive, self-effacing style that required attention to the dialogue and a responsiveness to the actual situation created on stage.

Ibsen's understanding of interior life makes his account of madness particularly of interest in so far as it addresses the phenomenology of madness, its explicit signs, origins and consequences. Ibsen's characters are carefully observed and some are drawn from real life. This aspect of Ibsen's writing, the relationship between his real life and his characterisation of the *dramatis personae* is another dimension to his art. We have knowledge of Ibsen's life, his friendships and relationships, such that the temptation to seek the models of his characters, to investigate the sources of his plots is often irresistible. Furthermore, Ibsen's male characters are as singular as any known to drama: Osvald Alving in *Ghosts*; Tomas Stockmann in *An Enemy of the People*; Arnold Rubek in *When We Dead Awaken*; John Rosmer in *Rosmersholm*; Halvard Solness in *The Master Builder*; and John Gabriel Stockman in *John Gabriel Borkman* all have intense inner life, driven by hidden conflicts or convictions. But, perhaps it is his female characters that are most singular. It is arguable that not since Euripides have female characters been created with as much sympathy. Hedda Gabler in *Hedda Gabler*; Helena Alving in *Ghosts*; Ellida Wangel in *The Lady From the Sea*; and Nora in *A Doll's House* all have resolve, even obstinacy, often in the face of odds.

Ibsen is described as having dealt with social issues of his day, but it is his understanding of psychology, his grasp of inner life, his pursuit of the truth of experience that continues to astonish today. It is this capacity to interpret and reveal that which is secretive and lurking in the shadows of the soul that make his plays of continuing relevance and importance. This fact, Ibsen's theatre of the mind, is also a window first on his conception of madness, second on how madness was understood in his day, and third on the uses of madness as a device in drama. Ibsen can be said to have domesticated drama if by 'domestication' we mean the normalisation of dramatic events. Ibsen was careful to give exact directions about the set, for example, in *Romersholm*, he instructed:

> 'The living-room at Romersholm, large, old-fashioned, and comfortable. Downstage against the right-hand wall is a tiled stove dressed with fresh birch-branches and wild flowers. Further back is a door. In the back wall, a folding door to the hall. In the left-hand wall, a window and in front of it a stand with flowers and plants. By the stove is a table with a sofa and easy chairs. All round the walls hang portraits, older or more recent, of clergy, officers, and government officials in uniform. The window stands open and so does the door to the hall and the outer door of the house. Outside can be seen an alley of tall old trees leading up to the house. It is a summer evening and the sun is down.'

(Ibsen, 1958: p. 29)

These directions are detailed almost to the point of fastidiousness. In essence, Ibsen is creating a particularly recognisable environment, a motif if you wish. The set was doing more than merely providing the physical space in which events are played. The physical space itself was speaking to the audience and mirroring the real world, a familiar everyday world in which the actors spoke in ordinary language much as people did on a daily basis. Davis (1992) argues that Ibsen 'made the events of his plays contemporary and placed them in homes with which his audience were familiar' (p. 26), thereby his plays 'have aroused intense interest and fierce and sustained controversy' (p. 26). The case that Davis is arguing is that audiences only partially identify with the characters in most plays because of a process of 'distancing' which is achieved by the characters being portrayed in an unfamiliar environment. Thus, Ibsen's plays intensify the identification process by emphasising the common ground shared by the characters in the play and the audience. To the extent that Ibsen portrays madness in his plays, by definition he also domesticates madness, making it more real, more actual, much more a possibility in the lives of the audience, thereby more threatening but also more understandable.

Ghosts and burden of the past

Ghosts was first published in December 1881. It is the story of a woman, Helena Alving, the widow of Captain Alving, who leaves her husband early in her marriage but is persuaded by Pastor Manders whom she loves to return home. She has a son Osvald who unbeknownst to her contracted congenital syphilis from his father. Davis (1992) has argued that the play deals with shackles of the past and that it is autobiographical. Ibsen's father was a bankrupt and this had forced the Ibsens, like the Alvings in the play, to move out of town to a house where they felt socially isolated and of inferior status. At the heart of the play is the secret of Captain Alving's dissolute life that had been kept concealed from Osvald.

The play turns on the recapitulation of Captain Alving's life in the life of his son. Helena Alving overhears her son making sexual advances to the maid-servant Regina, just as his father had done to Regina's mother. This replaying of the past in the present amplifies the tragic potential of the play for there is now the possibility of avoiding the inevitable tragic ending. The burden of the past is the 'ghosts' of the title. In this appreciation of the continuing influence of the past on the present, Ibsen anticipated Freud. Helena Alving says to Pastor Manders:

> I'm haunted by ghosts. When I heard Regina and Osvald out there, it was just as if there were ghosts before my very eyes. But I'm inclined to think that we're all ghosts, Pastor Manders; it's not only the things that we've inherited from our fathers and mothers that live on in us, but all sorts of dead ideas and old dead beliefs, and things of that sort. They're not actually alive in us, but they're rooted there all the same, and we can't rid ourselves of them. I've only to pick up a newspaper, and when I read it I seem to see ghosts gliding between the lines. I should think there must be ghosts all over the country – as countless as grains of sand. And we are, all of us, so pitifully afraid of the light.

> (Ibsen, 1964: p. 61, Act II)

In *Ghosts*, it is not only memory, not merely the re-enactment of past events, not even ideas and beliefs about how life ought to be lived that acted as ghosts, emerging and disturbing the ease of the present, but the stigmata of a deceased father's dissolute life passed on as a disease to the son. This is literally the sin of the father visited on the son in the form of congenital syphilis, notwithstanding the arguments about whether Ibsen misunderstood the nature and transmission mechanisms of congenital syphilis or not. This affliction is as much a social stigma as it is a symbol of potential madness. Osvald Alving is stricken by fear, shame, regret and anguish to the degree that the state he imagines is worse than death:

> My whole life ruined – irreparably ruined – and all through my own thoughtlessness
>
> It's so shameful to have thrown away my health and happiness – everything in the world – so thoughtlessly, so recklessly ... My future – my life itself
>
> It's so unspeakably loathsome ... Oh, if only it had been an ordinary fatal illness ... because I'm not afraid to die, although I'll like to live as long as I can
>
> But this is so horribly loathsome. To become like a helpless child again; to have to be fed; to have to – Oh, I can't speak of it.

> (Ibsen, 1964: p. 98, Act III)

In *Ghosts* as in *A Doll's House*, Ibsen created female characters who conceal the ugly core of their family life, the family secret, who protect their husbands and in doing so severely restrict their own potential. In Greek tragedy, the plays take place in public spaces shared by the community, and the tragic, violent outcomes are hidden from the audience's sight. In Ibsen the set's three sides create an ordinary home that is open to the view of the audience. In essence, the audience is invited in to experience what goes on behind closed doors. The shock for the audience was that despite the apparent respectability of the characters, what was hidden from view was unedifying. This caused shock and anger. Meyer (1967) notes:

> 'So explosive was the message of *A Doll's House* – that a marriage was not sacrosanct, that a man's authority in his home should go unchallenged, and that the prime duty of anyone was to find out who he or she really was and to become that person.'

> (p. 476)

In the preface to his short stories *Marriage*, Strindberg wrote:

> 'Marriage was revealed as being a far from divine institution, people stopped regarding it as an automatic provider of absolute bliss, and divorce between incompatible parties came at last to be accepted as conceivably justifiable.'

> (quoted in Meyer, 1967: p. 467)

As with *A Doll's House*, the reception of *Ghosts* was not warm to say the least. Hundreds of copies were returned to the publisher; it was not a book to keep at home. It attacked marriage, undermined the duty of a son to his father. It also referred to venereal disease indirectly but unmistakably, hinted that incest might be justifiable and defended free love. At the core of the play is congenital neurosyphilis, an acquired form of madness, and the symbolism is intensified by the double jeopardy of an acquired venereal disease and of madness. In *Ghosts*, madness is therefore only a symbolic device; we do not see it enacted, neither do we quite grasp the full implications. This was probably in deference to the sensitivities of the audience at the time.

In *Rosmersholm*, *The Master Builder*, and *Little Eyolf*, suicide, death of children, and permanent disability of a child respectively are the events that the characters have to adapt to. In these plays Ibsen shows his understanding of human emotions, of the inner life as it responds to extreme challenges. Although none of the characters are mad in the ordinary sense, melancholia, guilt, anger, vengeance and jealousy are all well drawn.

Suicide at Rosmersholm

Rosmersholm was published in November 1886. Ibsen had made some brief notes when he first started to conceive the play:

> '*He*, a refined, aristocratic character, who has switched to a liberal viewpoint and been ostracised by all his former friends and acquaintances. A widower; had been unhappily married to a half-mad melancholic who ended by drowning herself.
>
> '*She*, the governess of his two daughters, emancipated, hot-blooded, somewhat ruthless beneath a refined exterior. Is regarded by their acquaintances as the evil spirit of the house; an object of suspicion and gossip.'
>
> (in Meyer, 1967: p. 583)

This is a powerful play that mystified its first audiences. Edvard Brandes, a critic, was one of the few who understood it and praised it in a letter to Strindberg: 'unintelligible to the theatre public, mystical to the semi-educated, but crystal clear to anyone with a knowledge of modern psychology' (Meyer, 1967: p. 584).

John Rosmer's wife had died by suicide outside of the time of the play, yet this event dominates it. The madness in the play is out of sight but very much in mind. Ibsen's brief notes and first drafts differed from the finished work in that the Rosmers in the finished play were childless, and the woman from Ibsen's notes, Rebecca, is John's mother's carer. Early on in the play, there is a searching for why Beate Rosmer killed herself:

> KROLL   Well, tell me then, what do you really think was the primary cause of Beate's ending her own life?

ROSMER Can you have any doubt about it? Or, rather, can one ask the reasons for what a person does who is unhappy, ill, and not responsible?

.   .   .   .

ROSMER If the doctors had sometimes seen her in the state I so often saw her in, day and night, they wouldn't have doubted then.

.   .   .   .

ROSMER ...I've told you about that uncontrollable, fierce passion of hers – that she insisted I should meet. Oh, the horror she filled me with! And then, in her last years, her groundless and consuming passion of self-reproach.

KROLL Yes, when she had realised that she would be childless all her life.

(Ibsen, 1958: p. 60, Act II)

This desire to understand the motivation for suicide, as if understanding will make the process of acceptance easier, is the heartbeat of the play, driving the action forward and leading surreptitiously to the final scene when Rosmer and Rebecca West jointly die by suicide.

We learn that Beate Rosmer 'was very nearly insane', and wonder with Rosmer 'where are we to look for the immediate cause of her sick mind passing over into madness?' And, this searching after meaning continued:

REBECCA Do you think Mrs Rosmer was in her right mind when she wrote that letter to Mortensgaard?

MRS HELSKETH It's so queer about the mind, Miss. I don't think, you know, she was right off her head.

REBECCA But she seemed to go all to pieces when she realised she couldn't have any children. It was then that the madness broke out.

(pp. 83–84, Act III)

The question of the origin of Beate Rosmer's madness is never resolved but the play makes clear that madness has a cause, i.e. that it is not a sudden irruption into conscious life without understandable social antecedents. In *Ghosts* it is an unspeakable possibility that is worse than death and in *Rosmersholm* it is outside of the events of the play. In the former, even though madness is brought about by syphilis, it is the result of a dissolute life, and in the latter, madness is attributable to the lack of children, a biological affliction with social consequences. This treatment of madness off stage is reminiscent of the Greek tragedy where the madness is described forcefully but never enacted, never portrayed for the purview of the audience.

To understand *Rosmersholm*, to grasp the inner tension, the unexpressed but active passion, even corrosive energy in the interactions of the protagonists, Mrs Helsketh's pronouncement: 'In this house children have never been used to cry, as long as folks can remember … And there's another strange thing, too. When they grow up they never laugh, Never laugh, as long as they live' (Ibsen, 1958: p. 84, Act III), points at the repression of feeling in the Rosmer family and also the absence of laughter in the district as a whole, beginning at Rosmersholm and spreading like an infection. It is this denial of feeling that makes possible the multiple avoidance of the truth, the denial of love and lust, and the indirect communication that only half hints at things and is more eloquent in silence than in speech.

Rosmersholm is the end of Ibsen's social and political commentary and the beginning of his psychological plays. It is a bridge between both periods for it deals with the nature of political liberalism but treats the psychology of the protagonists with equal force.

Davis has discussed the richness of Ibsen's understanding of psychology (1992). He shows how family secrets are often central to Ibsen's plays and how the revelation of the hidden truth allowed Ibsen to examine the consequences of truth telling. This aspect of Ibsen modernises the core of the Oedipus story in which Oedipus' desire for self-knowledge harms him. In *An Enemy of the People*, Dr Stockmann informs the local community that the water in the baths, the source of the community's wealth, is poisoned. However, this news is met with hostility such that he is ostracised by the community and regarded as an enemy of the people. Stockmann is referred to as 'mad' for his insistence, his perseverance in the face of opposition and his obstinacy, even though he occupies the moral high ground. In *The Wild Duck*, Gregers Werle provokes doubt in Hjalmar Ekdal about the paternity of his daughter Hedvig. This destabilisation of the family leads to Hedvig's suicide. It is Gregers who is regarded as 'mad' in this play for his importunate and intrusive truth telling, what Ibsen refers to as 'acute inflammation of the conscience'.

When another of Ibsen's plays, *The Lady from the Sea*, was published in November 1888, it was not well received. One critic referred to it as 'from first to last a story of sickness, a bizarre psychological case history, the development of which taxes the action of the play' (Meyer, 1967: p. 624). It is true that Ellida Wangel's character is melancholic and in the grasp of mental conflict if not anguish. She is Dr Wangel's second wife and has not been accepted by his daughters. She has a past encounter yet to deal with and resolve. It is said of her, 'I shouldn't wonder a bit if she were to go mad on our hands some fine day … Didn't her mother go mad? She died mad, I know' (Ibsen, 1919: p. 218, Act II).

The nature of Ellida's malady is never made clear, just as Rosmer's wife's madness was never exactly clear. But we know that Ellida Wangel experienced visual hallucinations:

ELLIDA Yes. Sometimes, without the smallest warning, I suddenly see him stand bodily before me. Or rather a little to one side. He never looks at me; he is only there.

WANGEL   How does he appear to you?

ELLIDA   Just as I saw him last.

WANGEL   Ten years ago?

ELLIDA   Yes. Out at Bratthammer. I see his scarf-pin most distinctly of all, with a large, bluish-white pearl in it. That pearl is like a dead fish's eye. And it seems to glare at me.

WANGEL   Good God – ! You are more ill than I thought; more ill than you know yourself, Ellida.

(Ibsen, 1919: p. 240, Act II)

Ellida's melancholy is attributed to her distance from the sea, the sea being her natural home. The source and quality of this sorrow is explored:

ARNHOLM   …We have once for all taken the wrong turning and become land animals instead of sea animals. All things considered, I'm afraid it is too late now to rectify the error.

ELLIDA   Yes, that is the mournful truth. And I believe people have an instinctive feeling of it themselves – it haunts them like a secret sorrow and regret. Believe me, this lies at the very root of the melancholy of mankind. I am sure it does.

ARNHOLM   But my dear Mrs Wangel, – I have never noticed that people are so profoundly melancholy. I should say on the contrary, that most people take life cheerfully and lightly – with a great, calm, unconscious joy.

ELLIDA   Oh no, that is not so. That joy – it is just like our joy in the long, light summer days. It has in it the foreboding of the darkness to come. And this foreboding casts its shadow over the joy of mankind, – just as the driving scud casts its shadow over the fiord. There it lies all blue and shining; and then all of a sudden –

(p. 255, Act III)

Dr Wangel concludes:

Have you not noticed that the people who live out by the open sea are like a race apart? They seem almost to live the life of the sea itself. There is the surge of the sea – and its ebb and flow too – both in their thoughts and feelings. And they never bear transplantation. No, I should have thought of that before. It was a positive sin against Ellida to take her away from the sea and bring her here!

(p. 288, Act IV)

The Lady from the Sea is remarkable insofar as Ellida Wangel's affliction, her malady, was cured by her husband setting her free to choose to leave him. Having restored her freedom, her autonomy to choose, to will her own future, she opted to stay with him rather than leave with the stranger whose memory was haunting her. Ellida declared: 'But you have been a good physician for me. You found, – and you had the courage to use, – the right remedy – the only one that could help me' (Ibsen, 1919: p. 346, Act V).

These plays required a degree of self-knowledge and courage on the part of the audience. The psychological depths that Ibsen was plumbing were too close for comfort; the characters were ordinary folk, not set in a distant country or in a remote historical period. To imagine that one's wife was unhappy because of an unfulfilling marriage, that the respectable father and member of the community had a hidden life that was unsavoury, or that dishonesty and unreliability were both rife in public transactions, these truths were not easy to dramatise in the naturalistic mode that Ibsen chose without provoking a hostile response.

In *Little Eyolf* and *Hedda Gabler*, Ibsen once again examined the modern marriage. *Little Eyolf* focused on a child with a disability that resulted from parental error. This theme of disease (in *Ghosts*), death (in *The Master Builder*) or disability (in *Little Eyolf*) in a child occurring as a result of parental culpable action is one that Ibsen turned to again and again. It allowed him to consider the place of culpability, responsibility, guilt, blame and shame in modern life and in relationships. These emotions are set in the context of relationships in which emotions are restricted in amplitude, or in which there is a constriction of affect such that the relationships are emotionally barren, evoking iciness, a bleak or sterile landscape in which the characters are stultified and struggling for emotional contact. This scenario, of course, leaves quite a bit of room for growth and transformation.

In *Hedda Gabler*, Ibsen created a character that is at once powerful and repulsive: a woman whose sexual appetite was ample if not excessive. Hedda Gabler was wilful and demanded of life that it be lived according to her own designs. Her suicide was unexpected and the early critics thought that it was unconvincing. Such belief that suicide ought somehow to be foreseeable, comprehensible in the light of antecedent events is still prevalent now. Ibsen had himself worked on this basis in other plays. In *Ghosts*, Osvald Alving in the anticipation of his mental decline had a store of poison to hand, and this was perfectly comprehensible. In *Rosmersholm*, Beate Rosmer's suicide was a puzzle to be made intelligible and the double suicide of Rosmer and Rebecca West at the end, though not exactly unexpected, was symbolic even if a romanticised emblem of incorruptible love. Clearly, Ibsen had created the impression in previous plays that suicide was not an enigma; rather, it was causally or teleologically comprehensible. Hedda Gabler's suicide, however, was a defining end point of a character who was singular, who defined herself against others, not by moulding or adapting herself but by resistance and obstinacy. There is a sense here that Ibsen was now moving towards his final plays, working with ideas and abstractions rather than making a social commentary or even examining psychological depth.

Madness in *When We Dead Awaken*

December 1899 saw the publication of *When We Dead Awaken*, bringing to a close the remarkable contribution of Ibsen to the dramatic world and the 19th century. Meyer (1967) has called the play a 'theatre of the mind'. It is the story of an old sculptor, Arnold Rubek, who has achieved much fame at the expense of personal emotional satisfaction, of happiness. He is married to a younger woman and on return to Norway meets his former model, Irena, who is deranged. Rubek and Irena climb to the top of a cold mountain and are killed in an avalanche. The play works at several levels, as a straight narrative dramatising the last days of an artist who is reviewing his life. But as a play, it has much in common with Euripides' *The Bacchae*, in its use of symbols with which much is being transacted that means more than is expressed in the superficial words.

Irena is Ibsen's manifestly mad character. Her utterances are strange and cryptic but to a psychiatrist they are surprisingly true to life:

PROFESSOR RUBEK   Some of the strings of your being have broken.

IRENA   Surely that always happens when a young warm-blooded woman dies.

PROFESSOR RUBEK   Oh, Irena, these are only delusions – shake them off. You're alive, do you hear? Alive! Alive!

IRENA   For many years I was dead. They came and bound me – they laced my arms together behind my back, and lowered me into a tomb, with iron bars over the opening, and padded walls … so that no one on earth overhead should hear the shrieks from the tomb. But now, I'm beginning to rise – a little – from the dead.

(Ibsen, 1964: p. 244, Act I)

Côtard's syndrome was first described in 1882. Côtard wrote:

'I would suggest the name 'nihilistic delusions' (*délire de negations*) to describe the condition of the patients to whom Griesinger was referring, in whom the tendency towards negation is carried to its extreme. If they are asked their name or age, they have neither – where they were born? They were not born. Who were their father and mother? They have no father, mother, wife, or children. Have they a headache or pain in the stomach, nor any other part of the body? They have no head or stomach and some even have no body. If one shows them an object, a rose or some other flower they answer, 'that is not a rose, not a flower at all'. In some cases negation is total. Nothing exists any longer, not even themselves.'

(Quoted in Oyebode, 2008: p. 141)

Case histories describe instances where patients say very clearly and unambiguously that they are already 'dead and buried'. Whether Ibsen had come across such case reports or had simply invented a character with this condition is impossible to tell. Irena says: 'I gave you my soul – young and living. And since then I've been empty – soulless. That's why I died, Arnold' (Ibsen, 1964: p. 250, Act I).

Irena's madness has a comprehensible source. It tracks back to her role as a model for Rubek. For Rubek, she was a mere body not a woman with feelings and desires, and that relationship was noxious to her spirit, devouring her soul and thereby rendering her dead, empty of life. Between Rubek and Irena, the sculpture that emerged was their child, a marble statue, inert and cold, kept in a museum; a place Irena called a 'sepulchre'.

This is a tragic last play because it examines what the life of an artist is, sacrificed to art, and impoverished as a result, impoverished of rich personal relationships. The toxin is equally damaging to collaborators as it is to the artist. If this was Ibsen's final assessment of his life's work, it is dark, bleak and unremittingly gloomy. There were already hints in the preceding play *John Gabriel Borkman* that Ibsen's self-assessment tended on the dark, morbidly gloomy side.

The following exchange captures the mood of the loss of opportunity:

PROFESSOR RUBEK A summer night on the hillside. With you! Oh, Irena – that might have been our life. That's what we have thrown away, you and I.

IRENA We see the irreparable only when –

PROFESSOR RUBEK When – ?

IRENA When we dead awake.

PROFESSOR RUBEK What do we really see then?
IRENA We see that we have never lived.

(Ibsen, 1964: p. 278, Act 2)

References

Davis, D. R. (1992) *Scenes of Madness: A Psychiatrist at the Theatre*. Routledge.

Ibsen, H. (1919) *The Collected Works of Henrik Ibsen Volume IX*. Heinemann.

Ibsen, H. (1950) *Hedda Gabler and Other Plays* (transl. U. Ellis-Fermor). Penguin Books.

Ibsen, H. (1958) *The Master Builder and Other Plays* (transl. U. Ellis-Fermor). Penguin Books.

Ibsen, H. (1964) *Ghosts and Other Plays* (transl. P. Watts). Penguin Books.

Meyer, M. (1967) *Ibsen*. Penguin Books.

Oyebode, F. (2008) *Sims' Symptoms in the Mind: An Introduction to Descriptive Psychopathology*. Saunders Elsevier.

CHAPTER 5

Tennessee Williams and the theatre of the mind

Ibsen and his contemporaries, Strindberg and Chekhov, irrevocably altered the nature of drama by the use of ordinary colloquial language rather than the hieratic language of verse. They domesticated drama by situating it within recognisably ordinary homes and dressed the personages in the same attire as the audience, thereby eradicating the emotional distance between audience and actors. Ibsen in particular developed, explored and enriched the psychological dimension of drama. In *Ghosts, Little Eyolf, The Master Builder, Hedda Gabler, The Wild Duck, When We Dead Awaken*, and other plays he created strong, deep characters with intense and interesting inner lives.

Strindberg's contribution was to expand the setting from the sitting room to a kitchen in *Miss Julie* (first published in 1888). The journey from public space in classical Greek tragedy to parlour in Ibsen had finally led, perhaps inexorably, to the kitchen, an unglamorous, hidden but important place within all households. In *Miss Julie*, Strindberg by his own account gave his characters a 'multiplicity of motives' (1964: p. 94) and did not fix them into an inflexible mould but rather rendered them vacillating and unpredictable, as was suitable for modern characters. This was Strindberg's not-so-covert attack on his rival, Ibsen's approach to dramatic characters. Furthermore, drawing from real people, Strindberg demonstrated in *The Ghost Sonata* the potential of creating characters who were so out of the ordinary as to make Ibsen's realism something of the past and to point forward to a different kind of theatre – 'The Mummy' in *The Ghost Sonata* lived locked away in a cupboard and was regarded as mad. Finally, in Strindberg, realism was starting to give way to a different method of ensuring that audiences remained attentive and alive to the possibilities of drama.

It was this heritage that the American dramatists Tennessee Williams and Eugene O'Neill inherited. Between them they submitted their own individual personal histories to scrutiny and made of their own anguished, troubled early life experiences art that remains a masterly example of psychological examination and exposition.

In *The Glass Menagerie*, Tennessee Williams (1911–1983) describes Laura Wingfield thus:

'Amanda [Laura's mother] having failed to establish contact with reality, continues to live vitally in her illusions, but Laura's situation is even graver. A childhood illness has left her crippled, one leg slightly shorter than the other, and held in a brace. This defect need not be more than suggested on the stage. Stemming from this, Laura's separation increases till she is like a piece of her own glass collection, too exquisitely fragile to move from the shelf.'

(Williams, 2009: p. xv)

In *A Streetcar Named Desire*, Tennessee Williams created the character of Blanche DuBois, a Southern belle fallen on hard times trying to hang on to a facsimile of gentility, traditional values and grace, but failing and ending tragically mad.

Both Laura Wingfield and Blanche DuBois were drawn from Miss Rose, Tennessee Williams' sister who in 1937 had a prefrontal lobotomy and spent much of the rest of her life in asylums. Williams' wrote:

'But you don't know Miss Rose and you never will unless you come to know her through this 'thing', for Laura of *Menagerie* was like Miss Rose only in her inescapable 'difference', which that old female bobcat Amanda would not believe existed. And as I mentioned, you may know only a little bit more of her through 'Portrait of a Girl in Glass.'

(1972: p. 125)

Tennessee Williams fully understood the risks, the limitations of realism and perhaps also that theatre drawing from memory needed to avoid becoming a documentary, an enactment of prosaic day-to-day life without the poetry that transforms drama into something other than dull, repetitive life:

'Being a 'memory play', *The Glass Menagerie* can be presented with unusual freedom of convention. Because of its considerably delicate or tenuous material, atmospheric touches and subtleties of direction play a particularly important part. Expressionism and all other unconventional techniques in drama have only one valid aim, and that is a closer approach to truth. When a play employs unconventional techniques, it is not, or at least shouldn't be, trying to escape its responsibility of dealing with *reality* [my italics], or interpreting experience, but is actually or should be attempting to find a closer approach, a more penetrating and vivid expression of things as they are. The straight realistic play with its genuine Frigidaire and authentic ice-cubes, its characters who speak exactly as its audience speaks, corresponds to the academic landscape, and has the same virtue of a photographic likeness. Everyone should know nowadays the unimportance of the photographic art: that truth, life, or reality is an organic thing which the poetic imagination can represent or suggest, in essence only through transformation, through changing into other forms than those which merely present in appearance.'

(Williams, 2009: p. xvi)

The stain of difference

Tennessee Williams clearly indicated that it was Miss Rose's 'difference' that she shared with Laura Wingfield and Blanche DuBois. This 'difference' was marked out in Miss Rose's behaviour and language. This principle that the mad are different and that their difference is what marks them out has been exploited by dramatists since the Classical Greek tragedies as described in preceding chapters. What is novel in Tennessee Williams is his interpretation of what might constitute tragic difference and that we know his model.

Rose Williams is vividly described in the writer's *Memoirs* (1972). She was employed as a receptionist at a dental practice but only lasted a day, having fled and locked herself, weeping, into the lavatory. This singular event is altered in *The Glass Menagerie* such that Laura Wingfield pretends to have been attending a business college and typing instructor when she had actually been visiting the local museum and zoo. Rose was admitted to the State Asylum in Farmington in 1937 and later that year had a prefrontal lobotomy. There are accounts of her detached, indifferent reactions, when she took her brother around the ward at the asylum, and her matter-of-fact manner and response to questions about her environment. There are also accounts of her unusual beliefs, for example, that her grandfather was an impostor, an instance of Capgras syndrome, one of the delusional misidentification syndromes. She was also of a belief that she was the Queen of England and that she had a son, both being untrue. But, it was her original use of language that was most intriguing. In *Memoirs* (1972), Tennessee Williams reports several examples: 'Today the sun came up like a five-dollar gold piece!' (p. 126), 'Today we drove in town and I purchased Palmolive shampoo for my crowning glory' (p. 126), and 'It rained last night. The dead came down with the rain' (p. 127).

The stain of difference is in effect a brand, stigmata that render the character recognisably mad. Violent frenzy, folly, unusual dress or nakedness, unjustifiable beliefs and oddities of language are some of the marks that designate madness. In Tennessee Williams' hands, the marks of difference are drawn from a model that he knew well and also loved:

> 'I may have inadvertently omitted a good deal of material about the unusually close relations between Rose and me. Some perceptive critic of the theatre made the observation that the true theme of my work is 'incest'. My sister and I had a close relationship, quite unsullied by any carnal knowledge. As a matter of fact, we were rather shy of each other...And yet our love was, and is, the deepest in our lives and was, perhaps, very pertinent to our withdrawal from extrafamilial attachments.'

> (1972: p. 119–120)

The effect of this closeness and affection is that Tennessee Williams treats difference, madness, with understanding and sympathy. Yet, his characterisation works and is convincing. Laura Wingfield in *The Glass Menagerie* is not only emotionally fragile but also crippled. Tennessee Williams directs that this defect be merely suggested and not accentuated. Her brother Tom responds to their mother Amanda's comment that Laura is 'lovely and sweet and pretty' (Williams, 2009: p. 42, Scene 5) by saying, 'Laura seems all those things to you and me because she's ours and we love her. We don't even notice she's crippled any more' (p. 42).

In a later exchange Tom develops this idea further:

T O M   Laura is very different from other girls.

A M A N D A   I think the difference is all to her advantage.

T O M   Not quite all – in the eyes of others – strangers – she is terribly shy and lives in a world of her own and those things make her seem a little peculiar to people outside the house.

(p. 43)

The Glass Menagerie is an exploration of difference, the value, potency and valence of difference. Jim, the gentleman caller, knocks over one of Laura's glass pieces, the unicorn, and breaks it. The unicorn has been described as 'extinct in the modern world' (Williams, 2009: p. 74, Scene 7) and 'lonesome' (p. 75). It loses its horn when Jim knocks it over and Laura reacts by saying 'Now it is just like all other horses', and 'I'll just imagine he had an operation. The horn was removed to make him feel less – freakish! Now he will feel at home with the other horses, the ones that don't have horns…' (p. 77).

In a series of exchanges with Laura, Jim attempts to pin down the inherent value of difference:

[Pretty] in a very different way from anyone else. And all the nicer because of the difference, too…The different people are not like other people, but being different is nothing to be ashamed of. Because other people are not such wonderful people. They're one hundred times one thousand. You're one times one! They walk all over the earth. You just stay here. They're common as – weeds, but – you – well, you're – *Blue Roses*!

(p. 78)

This idea that what is singular and different, what stands out is preferable for being rarer argues against the notion that the unicorn might be 'lonesome' for being different. It also stands in contradistinction to the Chinese adage that 'it is the nail that stands out that is bashed in'. Hence, Laura's oddities of behaviour, her emotional fragility, hers and Rose's autism, their palpable difference are valorised, not devalued. It is also this singularity of temperament, of disposition and personality that a memorable dramatic character is composed of. It is in *A Streetcar Named*

Desire that Tennessee Williams achieves a fully developed character based upon his sister, where the character's difference is not the subject matter, rather it is their psychology, even psychopathology that counts and hence is dramatised.

Madness and illusion

In Cervantes' *Don Quixote*, illusion is a human phenomenon that colours our understanding of reality, and that allows life to be bearable. It is a truism that we do not have knowledge of things as they are, only as they appear to us. What is less obvious but equally important is the degree to which the observed and perceived world is imbued with and strongly influenced by our expectations. Quixote succumbs to the elementary illusion that 30 or 40 windmills are actually a race of giants whom he wishes to battle. But, at its most sophisticated, Quixote's existence also drew attention to subtler forms of illusion, the tendency to see beauty where none exists or to see virtue or ability in those close to us whom we love:

> 'It can happen that a man has an ugly, charmless son, and his love blindfolds him to prevent him from seeing the child's defects: on the contrary, he regards them as gifts and graces, and describes them to his friends as examples of wit and cleverness.'

> (Rutherford, 2000: p. 3)

Strictly speaking, illusion refers to a false perception, which arises as a misinterpretation of a real object. Typically, a chair might be perceived as a leopard that is poised to leap and attack the person looking at it. The nature of the perception is often determined by the emotional state and the expectancy generated by the situation. So, an anxious person who is fearful of an attack by a wild animal on their first visit to the Serengeti might misperceive a chair as a dangerous leopard. It is also not the case that illusions are characteristic of madness as they occur with great frequency in normal people and are not limited to individuals who are mentally unwell. The distortions of reality that are pathognomonic of madness are hallucinations and delusions. Nonetheless, illusions constitute a common dramatic mechanism for denoting madness: Heracles' (Hercules') frenzy and the killing of his children or Ajax and the slaughtering of sheep under the misapprehension that he was fighting an army are classical examples of the use of illusion as a device to signal madness and to excuse tragic conduct.

In literature and drama, illusion is at the heart of the narrative. In drama, particularly, illusion is centre stage, so to speak. The scene is a representation of something other than itself. The actors are acting a part that is distinct from their own lives. Thus, nothing is what it seems. Time is compressed, a sense of reality is suspended, and language, no matter how naturalistic, is formalised and rehearsed. Illusion is accentuated and fostered by the set, lighting, costume and stage direction. Similar to *Don Quixote*, *A Streetcar Named Desire* is about the capacity of the individual to live in an illusory world, a world that ignores the grim reality despite being aware of it. This is not the same as denial of the facts, nor is it the same as burying one's head in the sand. It is dipping in and out of the fact of reality – remaining aware of the decay and dilapidation of existence, of the pain and anguish that it causes, but yet, as Blanche DuBois, continuing to live to the rules and conventions of a different time, the mores of a dying culture. It requires breathtaking audacity to treat illusion as the central theme of a play since a play is itself an illusion. Yet, it is this task that Tennessee Williams sets himself.

In *A Streetcar Named Desire*, Tennessee Williams' stage directions aim at suggesting more than can be communicated by mere words, costume or set. He directs that lighting, colour and music contribute to the atmosphere, to the shaping of the illusion that the protagonists inhabit. Thus, there is a filmic atmosphere to the staging. At the beginning of the play, he directs that:

> 'It is first dark of an evening in May. The sky that shows round the dim white building is a peculiarly tender blue, almost turquoise, which invests the scene with a kind of lyricism and gracefully attenuates the atmosphere of decay.'

(Williams, 1984: p. 3)

Later, he continues:

> 'The poker players – STANLEY, STEVE, MITCH and PABLO – wear coloured shirts, solid blues, a purple, a red-and-white check, a light green, and they are men at the peak of their physical manhood, as coarse and direct and powerful as the primary colours.'

(p. 24)

These directions are aimed at influencing the expectations of the audience, affecting and manipulating their emotions and thereby their experience of reality, of the world. In essence, an illusory world is being created. But why is so much energy being expended to inaugurate this world? Blanche DuBois partially answers this question:

> I don't want realism...I'll tell you what I want. Magic! Yes, yes, magic! I try to give that to people. I misrepresent things to them. I don't tell truth, I tell what ought to be truth. And if that is sinful, let me be damned for it! – *Don't turn the light on!*

(p. 72, Scene IX)

In addition to the urge to create, at least in narration, a world that is better than the one we have, there is also the sheer fact that the physical world is prone to decay, to disintegration, and that the world imagined is immune from decay and reliable:

> A cultivated woman, a woman of intelligence and breeding, can enrich a man's life – immeasurably! I have those things to offer, and this doesn't take them away. Physical beauty is passing. A transitory possession. But, beauty of the mind and richness of the spirit and tenderness of the heart – and I have all of those things – aren't taken away, but grow! Increase with the years! How strange that I should be called a destitute woman! When I have all of these treasures locked in my heart. I think of myself as a very, very rich woman! But I have been foolish – casting my pearls before swine!

> (p. 78, Scene X)

In the end, this strategy of creating an illusory world, as a buffer to dampen down the impact of oppressive reality is insufficient to the task – Blanche succumbs and is committed to the asylum. What are the factors that undermine her emotional stability? The most vivid is, of course, the rape of her by Stanley, her brother-in-law and the refusal by her sister, Stella, to accept Blanche's account as true. This denial by Stella points at a different kind of illusion, one that is unmediated by insight and is thus unfruitful and unlikely to result in transformation or growth.

The other causes that appear to contribute a dynamic to Blanche's fragility are enumerated early in the play:

> I, I, I took the blows in my face and my body! All of those deaths! The long parade to the graveyard! Father, mother! Margaret, that dreadful way! So big with it, it couldn't be put in a coffin. But had to be burned like rubbish! You just came home in time for the funerals, Stella. And funerals are pretty compared to deaths. Funerals are quiet, but deaths – not always. Sometimes their breathing is hoarse, and sometimes it rattles, and sometimes they even cry out to you, 'Don't let me go!' Even the old, sometimes, say, 'Don't let me go.' As if you were able to stop them! But funerals are quiet, with pretty flowers.

> (Williams, 1984: p. 12, Scene I)

The multiple losses of loved ones, the responsibility of watching them die and tidying up the family affairs coupled with diminishing family resources appear to have created a fault in Blanche's defences that were finally broken by Stanley's assault. But all these events were dangerous and potentially fatal because she had suffered a much earlier loss of someone she loved and lost. When she fell in love with him, 'it was like you suddenly turned a blinding light on something that had always been half in shadow' (Williams, 1984; p. 56, Scene VI), and when he died, 'then the searchlight which had been turned on the world was turned off again and never for one moment since has there been any light that's stronger than this – kitchen – candle ...' (p. 57).

Blanche's arid inner life, the impoverished internal landscape caused her to have 'deep, sincere attachments' because 'sorrow makes for sincerity' (p. 29, Scene III). This sense of emptiness and desolation created the urgent need for 'many intimacies with strangers', 'for intimacies with strangers was I seemed able to fill my empty heart with' (p. 73, Scene IX).

Blanche's language in *Streetcar* is unlike what we have come to expect of language use that denotes madness. It is not the nonsensical language of mad Poor Tom in Shakespeare's *King Lear*, nor is it the deliberately allusive and cryptic language of Hamlet. If anything it is often lyrical, insightful, transparently direct and informative. Martin Meisel has argued that 'a principal burden on dramatic speech is characterological, to establish and particularise identity' (2007: p. 65). One can add that in Tennessee Williams' hands, language can also be the vehicle for exteriorising inner tension and conflict, for explaining and exploring the origin of anguish, and finally for establishing the hierarchy of moral worth in contrast to what might be superficially the case. Blanche DuBois reveals much more than she avoids. She communicates inner steel despite her frailty and fragility. Even though she succumbs in the end, she retains her dignity.

In the final scene, Blanche's removal to an asylum is itself symbolic of the power of illusion in swaying emotions. The entrance of the doctor and matron is directed as follows:

'The gravity of their profession is exaggerated – the unmistakable aura of the state institution with its cynical detachment.'

(Williams, 1984: p. 85, Scene XI)

At the end, the doctor

'becomes personalised. The unhuman quality goes. His voice is gentle and reassuring as he crosses to BLANCHE and crouches in front of her. As he speaks her name, her terror subsides a little. The lurid reflections fade from the walls, the inhuman cries and noises die out and her own hoarse crying is calmed.'

(p. 89)

The doctor refers to Blanche as Miss DuBois and this act of old world courtesy and his taking of her extended arm provokes Blanche to say 'Whoever you are – I have always depended on the kindness of strangers.' (Williams, 1984: p. 89, Scene XI)

Both *The Glass Menagerie* and *A Streetcar Named Desire* are situated within families. The characters and the plot are comprehensible within the family context, but it is in *Cat on a Hot Tin Roof* that Tennessee Williams achieves his best examination of family life. Ibsen had already shown the possibilities of theatre that took contemporary, modern families seriously. He had exposed the dark underside of middle-class manners and overtly correct behaviour. One of his tools was the family secret, which impelled behaviour, distorted emotions, and motivated tragic action. Tennessee Williams developed this further. In his own view:

> 'That play [*Cat on a Hot Tin Roof*] comes closest to being both a work of art and a work of craft. It is really very well put together, in my opinion, and all its characters are amusing and credible and touching. Also it adheres to the valuable edict of Aristotle that a tragedy must have unity of time and place and magnitude of theme.
>
> The set in *Cat* never changes and its running time is exactly the time of its action, meaning that one act, timewise follows directly upon the other, and I know of no other modern American play in which this is accomplished.'

(Williams, 1972: p. 168)

This assessment of *Cat* by Tennessee Williams highlights the play's importance in his oeuvre. The play also deals with alcoholism, a condition previously regarded as evidence of characterological weakness, as a deficiency of the will in the face of resistible desire, a sign of akrasia, but which in the modern period has been medicalised and is now regarded as a mental disorder. In the following section, I will discuss *Cat on a Hot Tin Roof* and Eugene O'Neill's *Long Day's Journey into Night*.

Old sorrow, written in tears and blood

The family in *Cat on a Hot Tin Roof* displays all its warts in public. It is a patently mercantile unit, with its members determined to exploit their positions and roles for financial advantage. The characters are manipulative, deceptive, dishonest, brash, vulgar and intent on triumphing against death, against each other, against fate. The drama is as far from the respectability of Ibsen's *A Doll's House* as one can get without losing sight of the fact that it is the same societal structural unit, the family that is being dramatised. Where Ibsen was exposing hypocrisy at the heart of bourgeois society, Tennessee Williams was showing us that the American family was exactly a mirror image of the unashamedly individualistic and aggressive culture where material gain at the expense of everything else was the norm. Winning was everything. Hence, Brick in *Cat on a Hot Tin Roof* is exceptional and unusual having bowed out of this race, taking refuge in drinking, and ending intoxicated and detached from life.

Tennessee Williams makes sure that we know that *Cat* is very close to his own experience:

> 'Of course it is a pity that so much of all creative work is so closely related to the personality of the one who does it.

It is sad and embarrassing and unattractive that those emotions that stir him deeply enough to demand expression, and to charge their expression with some measure of light and power, are nearly all rooted, however changed in their surface, in the particular and peculiar concerns of the artist himself, that special world, the passions and images of it that each of us weaves about him from birth to death, a web of monstrous complexity, spun forth at a speed that is incalculable to a length beyond measure, from the spider mouth of his singular perceptions.'

(Williams, 1976: p. 7)

Eugene O'Neill makes this point even more succinctly in the dedication of *Long Day's Journey into Night* to his wife, Carlotta:

'I give you the original script of this play of old sorrow, written in tears and blood. A sadly inappropriate gift, it would seem, for a day celebrating happiness. But you will understand. I mean it as a tribute to your love and tenderness which gave me the faith in love that enabled me to face my dead at last and write this play – write it with deep pity and understanding and forgiveness for all the haunted Tyrones.'

(O'Neill, 1966: p. 5)

Both *Cat on a Hot Tin Roof* and *Long Day's Journey into Night* are autobiographical. It can also be surmised that the act of writing, of creative art has a personal purpose to it that is other than the artistic product, in this case, the play that the audience sees. For Eugene O'Neill the writing allowed him to come to terms with his own family, to comprehend them and to forgive. But for the play to work it must be more than merely personal history. Tennessee Williams understood this well: '… Out of your personal lyricism, your sidewalk histrionics, something has to be created that will not only attract observers but participants in the performance' (Williams, 1976: p. 8).

There is therefore in this process, too, a desire to communicate, to attract observers, at least to please them if not to seek their sympathy. This urge to speak to strangers 'in the hushed twilight of orchestra and balcony sections of theatres than with individuals across a table' (Williams, 1976: p. 9) makes of drama a space in which the contents of the mind, a particular mind, are exposed to our scrutiny. Theatre, originally a communal space, in which the whole community acted without strict demarcation between spectator and actor, has evolved from this provenance through its domestication within a secluded and walled-off space, to a spectacle of the enactment of the inner workings of a single mind. Each member of the audience is addressed personally, individually, but in the real time in the company of others, mostly strangers to him.

Alcoholism in *Cat on a Hot Tin Roof* is a response to the loss, by death, of a friend. Drinking here produces detachment and is aimed at inducing inner peace, but does not achieve this unfailingly. Drinking has a compulsive dimension to it that drives Brick to consume alcohol continuously to the exclusion of other activities. In this regard, *Cat* is an accurate representation of alcohol dependence. Brick's alcoholism is an epiphenomenon; it stands in for the disguised and defended homoerotic relationship between Brick and his deceased friend and teammate Skipper. The terror of impending death impels the action of the play: denial of a fatal disease, the struggle for an inheritance between the two brothers and their wives, and the ongoing battle for dominance within a marriage between Big Daddy and Big Mama. Tennessee Williams makes clear that the aim of the play is not to identify and make obvious the solution to one man's psychological problems, namely Brick's alcoholism; rather it is 'to catch the true quality of experience in a group of people, that cloudy, flickering, evanescent – fiercely charged! – interplay of live human beings in the thundercloud of a common crisis' (Williams, 1976: p. 75). He concludes: 'Some mystery should be left in the revelation of character in a play, just as a great deal is always left in the revelation of character in life, even in one's own character to himself' (p. 75).

It is obvious from the above that Tennessee Williams himself regarded *Cat* as a play about the interaction between the characters, about the discovery of depth and ingenuity, of determination and strength in Margaret, for example, in response to her personal crisis in the play. In her grit and resolve to re-possess her husband, to overcome his rejection of her, and to do this without his assistance and against the odds finds expression thus: 'Oh you weak people, you weak, beautiful people! – who give up. – What you want is someone to – take hold of you. – Gently, gently with love!' (Williams, 1976: p. 105, Act III).

Eugene O'Neill's *Long Day's Journey into Night* has no strong character. It is also a play about addiction, albeit addiction to morphine rather than to alcohol. The play is a dramatisation of O'Neill's family: the Tyrones are the O'Neill's. Eugene O'Neill was born in 1888 to James O'Neill, an actor and his wife Ella Quinlan O'Neill. Their eldest son Jamie, who was ill with measles, disobeyed orders to say away from his younger brother Edmund, who then contracted measles and died. Even though Ella had not wished for any more children, she was persuaded to have another child. The result was Eugene. His mother became addicted to morphine because of the difficult birth. Both brothers thereafter suffered guilt: Jamie for having inadvertently been the cause of his younger brother's death and Eugene for having been born at all. It is this family tragedy that Eugene O'Neill fashions into a play. As with *Cat on a Hot Tin Roof*, there is a meaningful, understandable heart to the morphine addiction. It is as if for the playwright addiction must be psychologically comprehensible. Mary Tyrone says:

> I was so healthy before Edmund was born … There wasn't a nerve in my body … But bearing Edmund was the last straw. I was so sick afterwards, and

that ignorant quack of a cheap hotel doctor – All he knew was I was in pain. It was easy for him to stop the pain.

(O'Neill, 1966: Act 2, Scene 2)

She goes on:

The past is the present, isn't it? It's the future, too. We all try to lie out of that but life won't let us. I blame only myself. I swore after Eugene died I would never have another baby. I was to blame for his death. If I hadn't left him with my mother to join you on the road, because you wrote telling me you missed me and were so lonely, Jamie would never have been allowed, when he still had measles, to go in the baby's room. I've always believed Jamie did it on purpose. He was jealous of the baby. He hated him. Oh, I know Jamie was only seven, but he was never stupid. He'd been warned it might kill the baby. He knew. I've never been able to forgive him for that.

The choice of names for the brothers in the play is instructive. In real life, the oldest brother was Jamie, the middle brother who died was Edmund and the youngest brother was Eugene. In the play, the middle brother who died was Eugene, the eldest brother as in life is Jamie and the youngest brother is Edmund. Such choice of names suggests that Eugene wished he had been the middle brother who had died. This play is not simply drawn from life but follows the real life closely, allowing only for little reworking. In this respect, O'Neill differs from Tennessee Williams who maintained some distance from his personal material. For Williams, the personal was merely a source of his art, not the end in itself. Both O'Neill and Williams capture the role of self-disgust in the psychology of addiction, as well as the function of lying or, as Brick referred to it in *Cat on a Hot T in Roof*, mendacity in fuelling self-contempt and disgust.

Long Day's Journey into Night is a true theatre of the mind. It is a re-enactment of O'Neill's memory, a staging of the playwright's inner psychological conflicts for the audience to watch. There is no transformation in any of the characters, the transformative power of the play lies in helping O'Neill to work through his conflicts, his 'old sorrows' so that he finally came to feel 'deep pity and understanding and forgiveness' (1966: p. 5). Yet, it is a compelling spectacle that is a privilege to observe at close quarters; a family tragedy in which all the parties are locked into a role that appears inescapable from within. The dramatic irony is knowing that one of the brothers survived this pitiful situation with enough inner strength, with the steel to dramatise his trauma, his wounds, his pain, if you wish his death, for he is Eugene the brother who died. But he resurrected himself to write for us. That is the triumph of Eugene O'Neill.

References

Meisel, M. (2007) *How Plays Work*. Oxford University Press.
O'Neill, E. (1966) *Long Day's Journey into Night*. Jonathan Cape.

Rutherford, J. (transl.) (2000) *Cervantes: The Ingenious Hidalgo Don Quixote de la Mancha, Part 1*. Penguin Books.

Strindberg, A. (1964) *Strindberg Plays: 1 (The Father; Miss Julie; The Ghost Sonata)*. Methuen Drama.

Williams, T. (1972) *Memoirs*. New Directions Books.

Williams, T. (1976) *Cat on a Hot Tin Roof. The Milk Train Doesn't Stop Here Anymore. The Night of the Iguana*. Penguin Books.

Williams, T. (1984) *A Streetcar Named Desire*. Methuen Drama.

Williams, T. (2009) *The Glass Menagerie*. Modern Penguin Classics.

CHAPTER 6

Soyinka's theatre of the shadowlands

Madness is usually conceived as a behavioural or psychological deviancy manifest in an individual. Thus, theatrical representations depict mad individuals. Even though theatre is a space where the social is exhibited, mirrored, examined, commented upon and defined, mad acts occur as solitary, even singular events, within social contexts. The social context may provide the origins, the motivating urge of the mad behaviour or may make the aberrant action understandable, rendering that which superficially is inexplicable, comprehensible and therefore meaningful. Even where the insane act is apparently motiveless and ultimately meaningless, it is against the background of shared values and self-evident and coherent mores that the motiveless and incomprehensible is shown to be understandable.

Referring to the Classical Greek period, Edith Hall argues that: 'Gatherings of citizens took place often and routinely, usually in the open air, as at the theatre of Dionysius. These gatherings were an essential social mechanism in shaping group opinion' (2010: p. 60). In other words, the Greek audience were discussing and responding to the dramatic material that they had watched. It is easy to imagine that plays such as Euripides' *Medea* and Sophocles' *Antigone* where there is a direct appeal to the moral sensibility of the audience would have evoked much discussion, acting as stimulation to discover the boundaries of what is permissible and defining and guiding conduct. In addition, it is clear that the comedies, particularly Aristophanes' plays, were often written in response to specific political and social events, either with a view to influencing the course of public life or merely to draw attention to those events by speaking the truth to power acting as 'mirrors for princes'. These social and public aspects of the theatre are arguably present in Shakespeare and are definitely important in Ibsen's plays, especially in *An Enemy of the People* and *Pillars of the Community*. In his later plays, Ibsen concentrated on exploring individual psychology, granted, of an individual in the context of modernity. Where Ibsen adopted realism as his chosen dramatic method, Tennessee Williams, who as we have already seen also explored individual psychopathology, moved away from realism by amplifying the illusory and borrowing some of Brecht's techniques by using scene announcements or commentaries, for example a screen legend or a screen image, as a counter to what was happening on stage. He thus alienated the audience from the characters, precisely what Ibsen was attempting to avoid, allowing the audience to take a fresh perspective on drama. This move away from realism that had already begun with Strindberg culminated in two distinct approaches, Brecht's epic theatre and what Martin Esslin has termed 'the theatre of the absurd' (Esslin, 2001).

Brecht's epic theatre was developed as a reaction against dramatic theatre. For Brecht, dramatic theatre among other things relied on plot, involved the audience in the stage situation, and demanded a linear development of the drama, whereas epic theatre was narrative in form and turned the spectator into an observer, forcing him to make decisions, and utilised montages with each scene standing for itself. Brecht's claim was that:

> 'The spectator was no longer in any way allowed to submit to an experience uncritically (and without practical consequences) by means of simple empathy with the characters in a play. The production took the subject-matter and the incidents shown and put them through a process of *alienation: the alienation that is necessary to all understanding* [my italics]. When something seems 'the most obvious thing in the world' it means that any attempt to understand the world has been given up.'

> (Brecht, 1964: p. 71)

The theatre of the absurd is an independent movement employing other dramatic techniques but in many respects it is similar to Brecht's epic theatre as having anti-realism as its goal. Martin Esslin has argued that the theatre of the absurd:

> 'Cannot provoke the thoughtful attitude of detached social criticism that is Brecht's objective. It does not present its audience with sets of social facts and examples of political behaviour. It presents the audience with a picture of a disintegrating world that has lost its unifying principle, its meaning, its purpose – an absurd universe. What is the audience to make of this bewildering confrontation with a truly alienated world that, having lost its rational principle, has in the true sense of the word gone mad?'

> (2001: pp. 411–412)

It is the idea of a world gone mad, society that no longer has coherence of culture, of unifying religious belief, of structures that determine what the values and rules to live by are. Again, Martin Esslin refers to the fact that the theatre of the absurd 'Expresses man's endeavour to come to terms with the world in which he lives. It attempts to make him face up to the human condition as it really is, to free him from illusions that are bound to cause constant maladjustment and disappointment' (2001: p. 428).

There are a number of techniques and devices that are common to the theatre of the absurd. There is a devaluation of language, a drawing on the metaphorical power of concrete, objectified images that are poetic in their concision and symbolism. There is also the use of dream images, the absence of plots and characters as ordinarily understood, and the use of montages of scenes that are not necessarily linearly derived from the preceding scene.

It could be argued that the same kind of conditions that made the development of the theatre of the absurd possible also exist in African society, although these conditions have arisen for different reasons, impelled by forces distinct and equally pernicious to the human spirit. In the past 100 years African societies have undergone the most astonishing cultural and societal shifts – changes in religious beliefs, in the nature and hierarchies of power, in the roles of men and women, in self-concept and identity, and in the most rapid urbanisation imaginable. In effect, the 20th century was one of great transition. The consequence of these changes is as exactly as described by Martin Esslin:

> 'A world where it is impossible to know why it [the world] was created, what part man has been assigned in it, and what constitutes right and wrong actions, that a picture of the universe lacking all these clear-cut definitions appears deprived of sense and sanity, and tragically absurd.'

> (2001: p. 425)

However, in Africa the overt societal response has not been necessarily to reject religion, to become immersed in ennui or anomie, or to become dislocated both psychologically and culturally. Rather, there is ample evidence of deepening and strident religiosity, strengthened affiliation to ethnic groupings, and an optimism that is belied by the facts of everyday life. Yet, the dispossession, human wretchedness and the innumerable wars are tractable to the failure of politics. Flora Veit-Wild comments in her book *Writing Madness*: 'the political situation in Africa is so full of absurdities, monstrosities and grotesque aberrations that it demands a literary response reflecting the innermost madness of this very situation and the structures ruling it' (2006: p. 2).

Madness and specialists

Soyinka's *Madmen and Specialists* was first performed at the 1970 Playwrights' Workshop Conference at the Eugene O'Neill Theater Center, Waterford, Connecticut, USA. Along with *The Road*, it has been described as having:

> 'All the hallmarks of modern, avant-garde drama: plotlessness, or radical non-linearity of plot; protagonists who defy any simple or coherent categorisation in terms of who they are and what their motivations are; a dramaturgical

method which foregrounds language and other means of expression as artistic means of production and representation whose yield in terms of aesthetic, political or ethical impact cannot be taken for granted.'

(Jeyifo, 2004: p. 142)

Madmen and Specialists was first performed after the Nigerian civil war that lasted from 1967 to 1970 and in which an estimated 1 million people died. At the heart of the play is the idea of the insanity of the gross loss of life during that war, and during all wars. This is a play refracting through its prism the enormity of the loss of life, using poetry to depict the insanity of war. This is not a play that yields its meaning easily or ever. It communicates its meaning by evoking the absurdity of an aspect of life. The powerful central taboo that the play challenges in order to force its audience to grasp the repugnant nature of war is cannibalism. It is subversive of the complacency of people uninvolved in war. It also has centre stage a cohort of beggars, that is, a group that normally lives in the liminal spaces, at the very edge of society, seen but not fully apprehended. This is an inversion that prepares the audience for the ultimate inversion of values, the valorisation of a cannibal feast. It is as if Soyinka sought to create a drama that induced in the audience the selfsame disgust that he felt when confronted by the obscenity of a war in which large numbers pointlessly perished.

In the foreword to another play, *Opera Wonyosi*, Soyinka's adaptation of Brecht's *Threepenny Opera*, Soyinka set out his diagnosis of Nigeria in the 1970s:

'The Nigerian society which is portrayed, without one redeeming feature, is that oil-boom society of the seventies which every child knows too well. The crimes committed by a power-drunk soldiery against a cowed and defenceless people, resulting in further mutual brutalisation down the scale of power – these are the hard realities that hit every man, woman and child, irrespective of class as they stepped out into the street for work, school or other acts of daily amnesia.'

(Soyinka, 1980: p. 298)

And,

'What does the class conflict have to say – or even more relevantly, what did the class conflict have to say about the epidemic of ritual murder for the magical attainment of wealth? Of those syndicates which kidnapped and murdered victims of all classes in order to convert their vital organs to wealth talismans?'

(p. 299)

Soyinka concludes:

'Those of us who see no reason to present a utopian counter to the preponderant obscenities that daily assail our lives and, whose temporary relief is often one of "sick humour", will continue to press this line of confrontation by accurate and negative reflection, in the confidence that sooner or later, society will recognise itself in the projection and, with or without the benefit of "scientific" explications, be moved to act in its own overall self-interest.'

(pp. 299–300)

It is clear that Soyinka's answer to his critics for his purported lack of socialist class consciousness was to state his project as a mirroring of the body politic so that it can come to recognise itself, to awaken to insight and become aware of itself. *Madmen and Specialists* is dark and has an opaque manner of telling its story for it is devoid of overt statements. It works at a deeper level, influencing consciousness and self-knowledge as if beyond what words convey. The principal character, Old Man, and his coterie of followers, the beggars, work towards the crisis of the play, the attempted ritual murder and presumably ritual cannibalism of one of the other characters. Old Man is described by Bero, his son to Si Bero, his daughter:

BERO   He's a sick man. He's coming home to be cured.

SI BERO   Sick? Wounded?

BERO   Mind sickness. We must be kind to him.

SI BERO   How long, Bero? How long had he been sick?

BERO   Ever since he came out. Maybe the … suffering around him proved too much for him. His mind broke under the strain.

SI BERO   [*quietly*] How bad? Don't hide anything, Bero. How bad is he?

BERO   He started well. But of course we didn't know which way his mind was working. Madmen have such diabolical cunning. It was fortunate I had already proved myself. He was dangerous. Dangerous!

(Soyinka, 1980: p. 247)

It was probably best that Old Man was 'mad' since his later actions were so totally against all native bonds of human affiliation:

BERO   …We said amen with a straight face and sat down to eat. Then, afterwards…

SI BERO   Yes?

BERO   He told us. (*Pause. He laughs suddenly.*) But why not? Afterwards I said why not? What is one flesh from another? So I tried it again, just to be sure of myself. It was the first step to power you understand. Power in its purest sense. The end of inhibitions. The conquest of the weakness of your too human flesh with all its sentiment. So again, all to myself I said Amen to his grace.

(Soyinka, 1980: p. 252)

Soyinka employs many of the techniques of the theatre of the absurd but he brings to bear on his material devices drawn from Yoruba theatre. Martin Esslin has argued that the theatre of the absurd has developed from older forms including pure theatre, which derives its potency from the spectacle of juggling or miming. Here the distinction between spectator and audience becomes clear. Pure theatre requires only attention to spectacle. But Soyinka has inherited and deploys the techniques of the masquerade. Spectacle is everything here too but the visual object and the thing represented are one thing. The masquerade is not merely a symbol but both symbol and represented object. This fusion between the signified and signifier is even more apparent in how language operates. In poetry, words operate not only as vehicles of language, transmitting a message and communicating, but, in addition to this ordinary aspect of words, in poetry words also exist as objects in their own right, objects that have luminosity, shape, colour, mass and a fibrillar or filamentous texture. They are objects that are explosive to the ears or that caress or provoke by poking, etc. Words in poetry behave like any other artistic medium; they have a malleability or resistance that the poet explores for full effect. Words have a force also in the Yoruba tradition, a power that can be toxic and malevolent like a curse or that can be pure and beneficent like a prayer. In *Madmen and Specialists*, unlike the theatre of the absurd of Ionesco or Beckett where language is devalued, Soyinka's theatre elevates language, the incantatory dimension of words:

> OLD MAN   ...You cyst, you cyst, you splint in the arrow of arrogance, the dog in dogma, tic of a heretic, the tick in politics, the mock of democracy, the mar of marxism, a tic of the fanatic, the boo in Buddhism, the ham in Mohammed, the dash in the criss-cross of Christ, a dot on the i of ego an ass in the mass, the ash in ashram, a boot in kibbutz, the pee of priesthood, the peepee of perfect priesthood, oh how dare you raise your hindquarters you god of dogma and cast the scent of your existence on the lamp-post of Destiny you HOLE IN THE ZERO OF NOTHING!

> (Soyinka, 1980: p. 292)

The language of Old Man combines the language games and playfulness of madness with Soyinka's understanding of words as aural objects. In *The Road*, the main character, Professor, is in search of 'the word', a vague, indefinable goal but with all the transcendence of the search for enlightenment. The madness in *The Road* is that of the world that those at the margins of economic life inhabit. The play is set in a roadside shack and the protagonists are drivers and touts. The language is exuberant and lyrical. Soyinka succeeds in formalising for dramatic purpose the urban pidgin English and another newly emerging dialect that fuses the urban pidgin with an American-accented English with words that have leaked into local usage from Westerns. Soyinka achieves what is perhaps one of the memorable speeches in African theatre when Say Tokyo Kid, a truck driver shows that irrespective of one's trade, there is inherent pride and a sense of distinction, and a drive, an urge to power and status:

> You think a guy of timber is dead load. What you talking kid? You reckon you can handle a timber lorry like you drive your passenger truck. You wanna sit down and feel that dead load trying to take the steering from your hand. You kidding? There is a hundred spirits in every guy of timber trying to do you down cause you've trapped them in, see? There is a spirit in hell for every guy of timber. (*Feels around his neck and brings out a talisman on a string.*) You reckon a guy just goes and cuts down a guy of timber. You gorra do it proper man or you won't live to cut another log. Dead men tell no tales kid. Until that guy is sawn up and turned to a bench or table, the spirit guy is still struggling inside it, and I don't fool around with him see, cause if your home was cut down you sure gonna be real crazy with the guy who's done it.

> (Soyinka, 1973: pp. 171–172)

Say Tokyo Kid continues:

> That me kid. A guy gorra have his principles. I'm a right guy. I mean you just look arrit this way. If you gonna be killed by a car, you don't wanna be killed by a Volkswagen. You wanra Limousine, a Ponriac or something like that. Well thas my principle. Suppose you was to come and find me in the ditch one day with one of them timber guys on ma back. Now ain't it gonna be a disgrace if the guy was some kinda cheap, wretched firewood full of ants and borers. So when I carry a guy of timber, its gorra be the biggest. One or two. If it's one, it's gorra fill the whole lorry, no room even for the wedge. And high class timber kid. High class. Golden walnut. Obeche. Ironwood. Black Afara. Iroko. Ebony. Camwood. And the heartwood's gorra be sound. (*Thumps his chest.*) It's gorra have a solid beat like that. Like mahogany.

> (p. 172)

He concludes:

> Timber is ma line. You show me the wood and I'll tell you whar kinda insects gonna attack it, and I'll tell you how you take the skin off. And I'll tell you whar kinda spirit is gonna be chasing you when you cut it down. If you ain't gorra strong head kid, you can't drive no guy of timber.

> (p. 172)

What Soyinka shows is that these people living in shadows – in the shadowlands – are also people in full sense of the word, with all the living, thriving desire in their chests. But their world is one in which physical violence is prevalent, where the horizon is foreshortened, and their living is precarious as the manner of it. One of the men makes his living stripping vehicles involved in accidents of their spare parts but also stripping the corpses of their possessions. It is what drives people to such a manner of living Soyinka turned his attention to in his later works.

Soyinka wrote in two different registers in his response to this mad world of 20th-century Africa. The one register was hermetic, opaque and difficult, the other, also borrowing from the theatre of the absurd, especially Jean Genet and Alfred Jarry, was transparent, comical, incisive and pointedly political.

The play of giants

Having described the mad world of contemporary Africa, Soyinka set his sights on the leadership class, identifying the abnormality of mind that was the root cause of the world presented in *Madmen and Specialists* and *The Road*. In the preface to *A Play of Giants*, Soyinka wrote:

> 'No serious effort is made here to hide the identities of the real-life actors who have served as models for *A Play of Giants*. They are none other than: President for Life Macias Nguema (late) of Equitorial Guinea; Emperor for Life (ex) Jean-Baptiste Bokassa of the Central African Republic; Life President Mobutu Sese Koko etc., of Congo Kinshasa (just hanging on); and – the HERO OF HEROES in the person of Life President (ex) the Field-Marshal El-Haji Dr Idi Amin of Uganda, DSc, DSO, VC etc., etc., who still dreams, according to latest reports, of being recalled to be the Saviour of Uganda once again.'

> (Soyinka, 1999: p. 3)

Soyinka concludes:

> 'For now ... (*Enter brass band, ringmaster, up platforms, hoops, and trampolines.*) ... 'Ladies and gentlemen, we present ... a parade of miracle men ... (*Cracks whip.*) ... Giants, Dwarfs, Zombies, the Incredible Anthropophagi, the Original Genus Survivanticus, (alive and well in defiance of all scientific explanations) ... ladies and gentlemen ...'

> (1999: p. 9)

Soyinka is here using all the tricks of comedy and parody to put these immensely funny characters under the spotlight. They would be merely funny if it were not true that their actions have had real effects in the real world resulting in death and injury to individuals and also immense damage to national economies. The play is set in New York at the Bugaran Embassy to the United Nations, in a building across from the United Nations. It is an exposition of the nature of power and how power is allied to base desires or even to the primordial urges unleashed by madness.

> KAMINI   As you speak, I wish I am there by your side. A man comes to life, in the middle of battle, not so? He feel power beating through his blood, *like madness* [my italics].

> (Soyinka, 1999: p. 31)

KASCO   Ants, ants, what they understand? Gnawing away at the seat of power. Flies, flies, what they care anyway? Buzzing around the red meat of power. The red blood attracts them, but what they do with the meat? Nothing. They lay maggots, the meat fester. You shoo them away, they run, buzzing away like noisy, excited children. What they can do? Nothing. But you turn your back, they come back – bz, bz, bz, bz. Power is the strong wind that drive them away. When the wind fall, when the sail of power is no longer fill, they come back. So, is better to squash them the first time. Don't blow them away, no. Squash them the first time, then you are saved later trouble.

GUNEMA   Zombies. Turn them into zombies. Is better. Any fool can understand government, but power! *Amigos*, that is *privilegio*. To control the other man, or woman. Even for one minute. Not many people understand that. When you control from birth to death, when the other man and woman know, in thousands or millions – I control your destiny from this moment, from this consciousness till the end of your life, now that is power. Even the animal world understand power, even the insect world. I have studied the colonies of ants in my garden. I sit down and meditate and collect my power from the night, and I watch the insects. Is very useful. I am not sentimental.

TUBOUM   I like to see the fear in the eye of the other man. If he my enemy, it is satisfactory. But it does not matter. If friend, it is better still. Even total stranger. Because I see this man telling himself, Tuboum does not know me, I am nothing to him, so why should he do anything to harm me. But he is afraid, I know it. I can see it in his eyes. I walk into a village, nobody in this village has seen me before but, the moment I arrive, I and my striped leopards – the village head, his wives, the priest, the medicine man, they are afraid. Sometimes I ask what is this fear I see? Have they been discussing treason before my arrival? Have they been holding meetings with rebellious Shabira tribesmen? But I know this is not the case. My spies have reported nothing, and they are good. They are afraid, that's all. Barra Tuboum has brought fear into their midst.

GUNEMA   I read once in a book – I think the author is Don Guadajara – he write that power is an elixir, how? That is when I go into voodoo. With power of voodoo, I do many things, many things impossible for ordinary man but still, I know I do not taste this elixir. If I taste it, I know. I watch the execution of these *mesquinos* who think they want to take my power. Firing squad, hanging, the garrotte, but still I do not taste this elixir. I do my own execution, take over gun, pull lever to hang condemned man. I use the garrotte myself but still, I do not taste this elixir. I watch when my zombies torture lesser zombies, I love their cries of pain, the terror before the pain begins. With some I watch the strength becomes weakness like baby, strong man cry like woman and beg to be put to death instead of suffer. It give the sensation of power but still, I do not *taste* this elixir.

(pp. 68–69)

G U N E M A Ah, but it is possible. It happen finally. I tell you. It happen like this. I sentence one man to death who I suspect of plotting against me. While he is in condemned cell, his wife come to plead for him. She is waiting all day in the house and when I am going to dinner she rush through my guards and fling herself at my legs, I am sorry for her. So, I invite her to have dinner with my family. Well, I make long story short. I tell her what her husband has done, that he is an enemy of the state and that the tribunal is correct to sentence him to death. She cried and cried, I feel sorry for her but, justice is rigid span of power, it must not be bent. My wife she is silent, she knows she must not interfere in affairs of state. That night, after my family retire, I take her to bed. Perhaps she think by that I will reprieve her husband, I do not know. We did not discuss it. But, I take her hand, and she follow me to my private bedroom. When I make love to her, I taste it at last. It is strong taste on my tongue, my lips, my face, everywhere. It rush through my spine, soak through my skin and I recognise it for that elusive, overwhelming taste. Every night I made love to the woman, the same taste is there, nothing to compare with it. Nothing.

(p. 70)

Soyinka achieves an incredible psychopathology of power. Here is the perversion of power, not as an instrument of beneficence or good will. These characters use power as an end in itself. Sadism, eroticism and orgasmic pleasure aligned to power, paranoid anxiety kept in check by fear and terror in the other, and other perversities of emotional life accentuated and strained by sheer unadulterated power are on display here. There is a sense in which the power on display is mad. It is an exaggeration, almost nightmarish excess unmitigated by reality constraints. Except that this is drawn from life, hence the mad quality of the conversation between these 'miracle men'.

In *King Baabu*, Soyinka (2002), borrowing from Alfred Jarry's *Ubu Rex*, moves outwards from the individual maladies of the characters in *A Play of Giants* to satirising the madness of the inner sanctum of power, the malady that resides in the coterie, that is propelled by self-interest and greed. It is an exposition of the venal strain in human affairs, the susceptibility to folly and delusions of grandeur and entitlement, the corruptibility of innocence. It is as if the madness of the African situation, the visible perversion of governance, the loss of the natural and instinctive moral code that determined what is permissible and what is good, and the rise to prominence of deeply amoral individuals is in the final analysis down to a core of corruption at the centre of power. This then infects those around the centre of power. But the external manifestations are the wars, the misrule, the oppression of ordinary people, and these plays do not suggest solutions nor do they analyse the problem in any systematic manner. As Soyinka himself says:

'Those of us who see no reason to present a utopian counter to the preponderant obscenities that assail our lives and, whose temporary relief is often of sick "humour", will continue to press the line of confrontation by accurate and negative reflection, in the confidence that sooner or later, society will recognise itself in the projection and, with or without the benefit of "scientific" explications, be moved to act in its own overall self-interest... To suggest that the turning up of the maggot-infested underside of the compost heap is not a prerequisite of the land's transformation is the ultimate in dogmatic mind-closure. All evidence in the material world of theatre and society asserts the opposite.'

(Soyinka, 1980: p. 300)

References

Brecht, B. (1964) *On Theatre: The Development of an Aesthetic* (ed & transl. J. Willett). Methuen Drama.

Esslin, M. (2001) *The Theatre of the Absurd*. Methuen Drama.

Hall, E. (2010) *Greek Tragedy: Suffering under the Sun*. Oxford University Press.

Jeyifo, B. (2004) *Wole Soyinka*. Cambridge University Press.

Soyinka, W. (1973) *Collected Plays*. Oxford University Press.

Soyinka, W. (1980) *Six Plays: The Trials of Brother Jero/Jero's Metamorphosis/Camwood on the Leaves/Death and the King's Horseman/Madmen and Specialists/Opera Wonyosi*. Spectrum Books.

Soyinka, W. (1999) *Plays: 2. A Play of Giants; From Zia, With Love; A Scourge of Hyacinths; The Beatification of Area Boy*. Methuen Drama.

Soyinka, W. (2002) *King Baabu*. Methuen Drama.

Veit-Wild, F. (2006) *Writing Madness: Borderlines of the Body in African Literature*. James Currey.

CHAPTER 7

Sarah Kane: the self in fission

The self is usually conceived as singular, retaining its identity continuously over time and having a distinct boundary separating it from other objects and selves (beings) in the world. Furthermore, there is self-awareness of vitality and of activity. Now, these characteristic elements of the self are retained in all the dramatic characters that we have examined. The personalities may exhibit deviant, aberrant behaviour, they may be homicidal or violent, their behaviour may have been irrational in the sense that it failed to meet some criterion of logic and reason. Yet, the characters themselves are coherent and whole individuals. In Sarah Kane's works we come before a different kind of person, one that is in fission. Even the dramatic voices at one stage become disembodied and appear to be emanating from a self in disintegration.

The 20th century saw the emergence of individuals who appeared to have multiple personalities, a condition that challenges our natural intuitions about the unity of the self. The first of these cases was Miss Beauchamp, described by Morton Prince in 1905. Prince wrote:

> 'Miss Christine L. Beauchamp, the subject of this study, is a person in whom several personalities have become developed; that is to say, she may change personality from time to time, often from hour to hour, and with each change her character becomes transformed and her memories altered. In addition to the real, original or normal self, the self that was born and which was intended by nature to be, she may be anyone of the three persons. I say different, because, although making use of the same body, each nevertheless, has distinctly different character: a difference manifested by different trains of thought, by different views, and temperament, and by different acquisitive tastes, habits, experiences, and memories.'

> (p. 1)

Prince went further to say:

> 'no one secondary personality preserves the whole psychical life of the individual. The synthesis of the original consciousness known as the personal

ego is broken up, so to speak, and shorn of some of its memories, perceptions, acquisitions, or modes of reaction to the environment.'

(p. 3)

The emergence in the empirical world of these kinds of cases in the 20th century can be said to have been anticipated by David Hume (1740) in *A Treatise of Human Nature*: 'what we call mind is nothing but a heap or collection of different perceptions, united together by certain relations, and suppos'd, tho' falsely, to be endowed with a perfect simplicity and identity' (in Norton & Norton, 2000: p. 207).

Hume concluded that 'the identity, which we ascribe to the mind of man, is only a fictitious one, and of a like kind with that which we ascribe to vegetable and animal bodies' (p. 259). This conceptualisation of the self characterised the unity and identity of the self as illusory. In other words, the Humean self has the characteristics evinced by individuals afflicted by multiple personality disorder – it is marked by an absence of unity or identity. Sarah Kane's theatre is natural and comprehensible within this compass. What is remarkable is that not more dramatists have taken the turn that Kane took. After all, creative writing, fiction and drama involve the invention of disparate characters whose origin is in the imagination of the author, that is, in the inner life, the psychology of the author. Yet, there is no question that the author loses his objectivity, his discrete identity. It is not even as though the process of writing, of authoring somehow cleaves the simplicity and unity of self. Or, that a weakness in the integrity is itself the motivating force, the source of the capacity to draw vivid characters and to infuse them with life, with memorable biography, temperament and comprehensible action. The reverse is more likely, that a coherent and integrated sense of self is a prerequisite for the creation of successful characterisation in literature.

Borges (1964) in his essay on Shakespeare wrote:

'There was no one in him; behind his face (which even through the bad paintings of those times resembles no other) and his words, which were copious, fantastic and stormy, there was only a bit of coldness, a dream dreamt by no one ... No one has ever been so many men as this man.'

(pp. 284–285)

Borges examined the nature of Shakespeare's identity and suggests that Shakespeare's fertile imagination for manifold dramatic characters was a mask for someone who was empty, who lacked a central core, hence Shakespeare's imagined statement: 'I who have been so many men in vain want to be one and myself' (Borges, 1964: p. 285).

There is no empirical evidence to support the contention that successful dramatists are any more emotionally or psychologically empty than anyone else. Nor is there any evidence that the richness of imaginative life reflects an impoverishment of the constitutive aspects of the self. The Portuguese poet Fernando Pessoa wrote under several pseudonyms or as is now described heteronyms including Alberto Caeiro, Ricardo Reis, Alvaro de Campos, Alexander Search, and under his own name. These heteronymous authors wrote in a defined style, were coherent and consistent in their poetic concerns, their diction and the scope of their poetry. If there was anyone emblematic of the supposed fragmentation in the human psyche in the 20th century, it was Fernando Pessoa. There is no evidence that Pessoa was other than an individual with a coherent self, although the writings and the fullness of the biography of the heteronymous authors superficially belie this fact. Pessoa's case is different from Sarah Kane's in that Sarah Kane's dramatic voices changed shape over the course of her short writing life, becoming fragmentary and disembodied and with the quality of inner speech or of verbal hallucinations in her later plays. The fact that Sarah Kane had a history of mental illness and was afflicted by recurrent psychotic depression raises the possibility that she drew inspiration from personal experience of abnormal phenomena. It also means that although artistic opinion may describe progression of talent over the course of her life, the changes in inflection of the authorial voice can certainly be mapped to a worsening course of mental illness and may indeed represent evidence of mental disintegration.

In Sarah Kane, therefore, drama has travelled the course from hidden but described madness of the characters in Greek tragedies to the focal and exposed inner workings of a deranged, disintegrating mind. These are polar opposites. Indeed, in Sarah Kane's works inner life and the theatrical space have coalesced to form a singular, imagined space into which the audience is immersed for better or worse. At the end, close to Kane's death by suicide, the characters, if they could be called that, have become nameless, anonymous embodied voices. These are fragments of her internal speech projected on stage for the audience to hear.

Reality in *Blasted*

Blasted was first produced by the Royal Court in January 1995. The play opens with the two protagonists, Ian and Cate entering a hotel in Leeds. David Greig (2001) in his introduction to Sarah Kane's *Complete Plays*, wrote of *Blasted*:

> 'Almost from the play's first words...there is an uneasy awareness that this play is not behaving itself. Ian's behaviour and language are unpleasant, repulsive even, and yet nothing in the writing is condemning him. No authorial voice is leading us to safety. As the play progresses, the moral unease grows until the scene finally changes, and we learn that, during the night, Ian has

raped Cate. Shortly afterwards, there is a knock on the hotel room door and, in the play's most daring moment, a soldier enters, apparently from nowhere, and brings in with him the terrifying fragments of a world blown apart by violence. It is as though the act of rape, which blasts the inner world of both victim and perpetrator, has also destroyed the world outside the room. The play's form begins to fragment. Its structure seems to buckle under weight of the violent forces it has unleashed. The time frame condenses; a scene that begins in spring ends in summer. The dialogue erodes, becoming sparse. The scenes are presented in smaller and smaller fragments until they are a series of snapshots: images of Ian, all the structures of his life destroyed, reduced to his base essence – a human being, weeping, shitting, lonely, broken, dying and, in the play's final moments, comforted.'

(pp. ix–x)

Blasted has all the hallmarks of the theatre of the absurd: language is devalued to the degree that the uttered words are banal, terse, and the exchanges are precise and unexceptional; the actions lack apparent motivation; the events are unpredictable and outside the boundaries of rational experience or of reasonable expectations; and the characterisation is in flux. As Martin Esslin (2001) put it in relation to the theatre of the absurd in general, 'We are confronted with a projection of a psychological reality and with human archetypes shrouded in mystery' (p. 417).

Like Harold Pinter, Sarah Kane strips down the dramatic encounter to a confrontation between two people, in this case Ian and Cate. We know little about their antecedents. This is a Pinteresque world:

'Apart from any other consideration, we are faced with the immense difficulty, if not the impossibility, of verifying the past. I don't mean merely years ago, but yesterday, this morning. What took place, what was the nature of what took place, what happened? If one can speak of the difficulty of knowing what in fact took place yesterday, one can I think treat the present in the same way…We will all interpret a common experience quite differently, though we prefer to subscribe to the view that there's a shred common ground, a known ground. I think there's a shared common ground all right, but it's more like a quicksand. Because "reality" is quite a strong firm word we tend to think, or to hope, that the state to which it refers is equally firm, settled and unequivocal. It doesn't seem to be, and in my opinion, it's no worse or better for that.'

(Pinter, 1991: pp. ix–x)

In Pinter as in Kane, the audience have to work to interpret what is going on. Nothing can be taken for granted. Even though language is reduced to the barest, leanest dialogue, it is still ambiguous and pregnant with multiple layers of meaning. Pinter, in *The Dumb Waiter*, creates a tense, dark, funny and dangerous world that is full of foreboding. In *The Hothouse*, set in an asylum, the action is inexplicable and progresses to violence and multiple murder. Sarah Kane in *Blasted* borrows from these motifs and atmosphere.

However, in the choice of language, the use of brutal images and shifts in action that rely on *quasi* dream-like images, she is different from Pinter.

In the essay 'Writing for the theatre', quoted above, Pinter refers to the 'quicksand' that is reality. Reality is by definition an issue for drama. Theatre is a space where the author's imagination is given life, projected for all to see. It is a make-believe world that aims for reality or in aiming against reality, points up the nature of reality. Ibsen's theatre uses realism as a tool to portray the Norway of his day. Nonetheless, his picture of middle-class Norway showed that what was projected as real was often illusory, hiding a reality that belied the respectable front that was projected for all to see. Tennessee Williams approached the subject in a different way. He showed that the internal world of the protagonists and by extension of the audience dictated how the characters saw the world and this was often at variance with how the world really was. Pinter looked at this issue from a different standpoint, that of a late 20th-century individual whose sensibility had been influenced by and had adjusted to the transitory nature of human relationships, their nebulous and indefinable quality. Right up to the beginning of the 20th century, relationships were determined by roles, kinship, and tribal affiliation. By the end of the 20th century it was no longer easy to predict with confidence the relationship between any two people observed walking down the street or conversing in a café. Hence, Pinter's plays confront the audience with dramas in which the narrative between the characters in the drama was unpredictable, if not full of tension and foreboding. The audience could make no assumptions about the relationship between the characters. In essence, Pinter's plays undermine our sense of reality. This is relevant for psychiatrists at many levels. The patient's encounter with the psychiatrist in the clinic is full of risk. The roles and relationships are not as easy to define as they might have been at the end of the 19th century, when psychiatry as we know it today first emerged. What is expected of both parties is ambiguous. The encounter can be experienced as threatening and potentially treacherous. Pinter's plays seek to capture the opacity of relationships, the potential for misunderstanding, the terror in the underbelly of all social encounters. Second, the patient's mental state infuses the encounter in the clinic with colour and tone, with expectations that are determined by psychopathology. Again, Pinter deals with the potential for paranoid interpretation in social encounters. In Pinter, what at first sight seems transparent and socially explicable can turn rapidly into perversity.

The Italian dramatist Luigi Pirandello's (1867–1936) opus was concerned exclusively with the question of the nature of reality. Pirandello's *Six Characters in Search of an Author*, *All for the Best* and *Henry IV* all deal with this subject in different ways. In *Six Characters in Search of an Author*, Pirandello explores the reality of the stage, dissecting out how the characters in the text differ from the actors who take on roles and bring the characters to life on stage. Pirandello emphasised the unvarying reality of the characters, their eternal quality and presence, waiting to be picked up night after night and enacted. Even more intriguing is their independent existence:

> 'I can only say that, having in no way searched them out, I found myself confronted by six living, palpable, audibly breathing human beings: the same six characters you now see upon the stage. They stood before me waiting, each one nursing his own particular torment, bound together by the mode of their birth and the intertwining of their fortunes, waiting for me to usher them into the world of art and make of their persons, their passions and their adventures a novel or drama, or at least a short story. They had been born alive and they were asking to live.'

(Pirandello, 1988: p. xiii)

In *All for the Best*, Pirandello showed how the same facts and behaviour in the light of changes in background assumptions alter understanding, meaning, and attitudes to the characters. The principal character discovers that his daughter is in fact not his, but the product of his deceased wife's adulterous affair and that he is the only one not to have known this. His continuing devotion to his deceased wife had previously provoked derision and contempt but in the light of the revelation that he was not aware of her affair provoked admiration. But the character's own self-concept changed dramatically. For Pirandello, meaning is determined by context, hence reality is not invariant but fluid and open to challenge and conflicting interpretation. In *Henry IV*, Pirandello dealt with the nature of madness. The principal character believes that he is Henry IV and his relatives humour him by creating a salon, furnished and decorated in the style of the throne room of Henry IV, and hence sustain his delusional belief. He recovers, but continues to pretend to be mad. Here we have differences in psychological reality masked by apparent similitude of behaviour despite this difference. Pirandello argued that:

> 'And while the sociologist describes social life as it presents itself to external observation, the humorist, being a man of exceptional intuition, shows – nay, reveals – that appearances are one thing and the consciousness of the people concerned, in its inner sense, another. And yet they "lie psychologically" even as they "lie socially". And this lying to ourselves – living, as we do, on the surface and not in the depths of our being – is a result of the social lying. The mind that gives back its own reflection is a solitary mind, but our internal solitude is never so great that suggestions from the communal life do not break in upon it with all the fictions and transferences which characterize them.'

(Quoted in Bentley, 1952: p. xiv)

This is the subject of Pinter's *Betrayal*, a play that opens in 1977 on a scene between two people we later discover have betrayed their respective spouses and closes in 1968 when the betrayal commenced. Things are not what they seem at the outset and only the past casts the right intensity of light to give meaning to the present. That meaning is determined by nuance of language use in the dialogue. It is not merely sexual betrayal that's at stake but how language itself betrays what is hidden, so that multiple layers of betrayal can coexist to the degree that it becomes difficult to identify who is doing the betraying and who is being betrayed, and whether language too is betraying the characters' thoughts. Again, the quicksand of reality is held up to the audience's gaze. This is also the subject of Shakespeare's *Othello*.

To return to Sarah Kane, in *Blasted* there is a shift from the syntax of objective reality to that of the imaginary world of dreams and hallucinations: a hotel room transforms into a war zone abruptly and without any preliminary mediation. Shifts in the structure of reality are part of the features of theatre of the absurd. Eugene Ionesco, for example, in *Rhinoceros* (2000), creates a world in which people gradually turn into rhinoceroses. Here, the boundaries of what is real are extended to include the possibility of human beings turning into animals. There is a sense in which Ionesco is using 'rhinoceros' as a metaphor, a concrete poetic image rendered live on stage in order to communicate an idea as if it were an objective fact in the real world. Sarah Kane's approach is different yet again: there is elision from one mode of experiencing the world to another without interruption, both inflecting on the meaning of the other. Sexual rape in this manner of experiencing reality is not merely akin to (civil) war but is war. It is the same impulse to violence, the urge to subjugate and triumph over another that is the substrate for sexual violence. The absence of overt structure and coherence to the narrative drive as the play progresses and the predominance of basic animal behaviour hints at deeper levels of consciousness, formless yet meaningful connections between disparate elements, as in dreams or delirium. In other words, Sarah Kane is utilising the resources of poetry, the apposition of disparate elements, to accentuate, exaggerate, adumbrate. The effect is subliminal, escaping rational censorship, deepening understanding and altering perspective in subversive ways. Yet, there is always the question whether the meaning attributed is genuine and intended or whether given the abruptness of syntax and the disintegration of form, the author may have lost control of the material, that the elemental subject matter may have overwhelmed the artistic, creative resources of Sarah Kane.

Inner speech and dramatic voice

In *Family Voices*, Pinter (1993) identified his characters merely as Voice 1, Voice 2 and Voice 3. Voice 1 is recognisable to the psychiatrist as probably someone suffering or recovering from psychosis. The language exhibits some of the tendencies typical of abnormalities of thinking processes and of speech:

This is the only room in this house where you can pick up a caravanserai to all points West. Compris? Comprende? Get me? Are you prepared to follow me down the mountain? Look at me? My name's Withers. I'm there or thereabouts. Follow? Embargo on all duff terminology. With me? Embargo on all things redundant. All areas in that connection verboten. You're in a diseaseridden land, boxer. Keep your weight on all the left feet you can lay your hands on. Keep dancing. The old foxtrot is the classical response but that's not the response I'm talking about. Nor am I talking about the other response. Up the slaves. Get me? This is a place of creatures, up and down stairs. Creatures of the rhythmic splits, the rhythmic sideswipes, the rums and roulettes, the macaroni tatters, the dumplings in jam mayonnaise, a catapulting ordure of gross and ramshackle shenanigans, openended paraphernalia. Follow me? It all adds up. It's before you and behind you. I'm the only saviour of the grace you find yourself wanting in. Mind how you go. Look sharp. Get my drift? Don't let it get too mouldy. Watch the mould. Get the feel of it, sonny, get the density.

(Pinter, 1993: p. 142–143)

In this speech a central determining tendency, that is, the goal of speech, is absent or not apparent. Speech progresses by the shifts occasioned by the acoustic aspects, or by immediate conceptual triggers in preceding clauses or suggested by features in the physical world. Hence, the fragility of the logical links between clauses and sentences, what psychiatrists would term a loss of association between concepts that results in disorder of the form of thought. *Family Voices* is also remarkable for the fact that the voices are not in dialogue but in simultaneous monologue. And there is tension and poignancy created and exacerbated by the apparent lack of communication between three people who we take to be relatives. Harold Pinter's *Family Voices* and *Landscape* presage Sarah Kane.

Sarah Kane in *Crave* (Kane, 2001) worked with four voices, identified simply as 'C', 'M', 'B', and 'A'. The voices have no unifying narrative thrust and there is neither overt characterisation nor context. As Greig (2001) put it:

'The overwhelming impression is that the four voices are, in fact, voices from within and without one individual life, yet the stage is occupied by four physically real bodies … The play's form, and this central, single image – four different bodies occupying one life – combine to evoke the powerful sense of a self fragmented.'

(p. xiv)

This idea of a fragmented self, a fissile self, split into four segments embodied in four physical bodies is the direct opposite of multiple personality disorder where the fragmented self, perforce, inhabits the singular body of the individual in question and has to make do with discrete biographies, personalities, voices and attitudes to communicate a sense of a multitude. In *Crave*, Sarah Kane achieves the impossible; she renders visible the fragmented self, yet retaining the anonymity of these fragments by identifying them simply with alphabets. These disparate selves are at once the inner speech of Sarah Kane, captured and transcribed for the theatre. It is also quite possible to imagine the voices as heard by her, as verbal/ auditory hallucinations that she records and transcribes for the audience. There is no distinction to be made between inner speech and auditory hallucinations, except that the hallucination is experienced as alien and other, and sometimes formally identified as this or that person. On the other hand, inner speech is within inner subjective space and is owned by the person as intrinsic to their being. Personal experience of auditory hallucinations may make it more readily apparent that these voices can be recast as characters in a play since the voices have that quality of being alien and objective to the individual who experiences them.

The utterances in *Crave* are dark, desolate, and devoid of hope though seeking love. These are statements that come straight out of psychiatric clinics:

> I'm evil, I'm damaged, and no one can save me
> Death is an option
> I disgust myself
> I am so tired
> Filled with emptiness
> I feel nothing, nothing. I feel nothing
> Whenever I look really close at something, it swarms with white larvae
> I open my mouth and I too am full of them, crawling down my throat.

(Kane, 2001: pp. 173–175)

These utterances point at Sarah Kane's intimate understanding of mental anguish and at her use of her personal experience as a source of artistic material. It is in her last play, *4:48 Psychosis* that she exploits her own experiences most overtly, mining her own anguish and disturbing experiences for material for her art.

Monologue of disquiet

Greig (2001) has argued that *4:48 Psychosis* 'describes the internal landscape of a suicidal psychosis' (p. xiv). It is pitiless, unrelenting in its excavation of the troubled mind:

> '*4.48 Psychosis* is a report from a region of the mind most of us hope never to visit but from which many people cannot escape. Those trapped there are normally rendered voiceless by their condition. That the play was written whilst suffering from depression, which is a destructive rather than a creative condition, was an act of generosity by the author. That the play is artistically successful is positively heroic.'

(Greig, 2001: p. xvii)

The language of *4:48 Psychosis* is poetic. Sarah Kane's language hitherto had been terse, precise and seemingly functional. Here it is lyrical, direct and compelling. It is reasonable to ask: in what way is this a play and not a long poem? It is the words that are on display, the words which by their physicality, their acoustic characteristics, dominate the stage. Here, the stage is the author's own mind laid open and visible to the audience. Instead of personalities treading the board, declaiming and acting, it is the words that are cast in the place of actors. Indeed, it is perfectly possible for the words to emanate from the walls of an empty stage and they would remain compelling and urgent. The misery, the intense and dense darkness, the revealed bleakness and the rhythmic pulse of the words, bare and rich as they are, determine and motivate the audience's emotions. Take for example:

> I am sad
> I feel that the future is hopeless and that things cannot improve
> I am bored and dissatisfied with everything
> I am a complete failure as a person
> I am guilty, I am being punished
> I would like to kill myself
> I used to be able to cry but now I am beyond tears
> I have lost interest in other people
> I can't make decisions
> I can't eat
> I can't sleep
> I can't think
> I cannot overcome my loneliness, my fear, my disgust
> I am fat
> I cannot write
> I cannot love
> My brother is dying, my lover is dying, I am killing them both
> I am charging towards my death
> I am terrified of medication
> I cannot make love
> I cannot fuck
> I cannot be alone
> I cannot be with others
> My hips are too big
> I dislike my genitals.

(Kane, 2001: pp. 206–207)

This is not confessional writing in the ordinary sense of the word. No secret acts demanding confession, remorse or restitution are being described. Yet it is confessional in that the list, the litany, emerges from the depths of being and is held up to scrutiny. The list reveals the nature of the intimate transaction that occurs within psychiatric clinic and how this, in Sarah Kane's hands, is turned into art. When the voice tells us 'I have become so depressed by the fact of my mortality that I have decided to commit suicide' (p. 207) and we are aware that the author did commit suicide, the author's suicide outside of theatrical time becomes part of the drama, for it both infects and inflects the drama with despair and tragedy.

The play is called *4:48 Psychosis*, because this was the time, early in the morning, when Sarah Kane in her final depressive episode, her final and fatal episode, would wake up to the horror of her situation. Early morning wakening is a typical, some would say, diagnostic feature of melancholia.

The theatre is a place of honesty but the represented world is fictive not real. The audience do not come to see a real knife plunged into a real chest with real blood gushing. Luigi Pirandello understood this point very well. In *Six Characters in Search of an Author*, Pirandello has the boy (a character) die and it is impossible to tell whether he has really died or whether it is make-believe. The point that Pirandello wants to emphasise is that characters can die, that is their reality and their nature, but the actors are only portraying a character and live to play the part another night. *4:48 Psychosis* straddles this divide between character and actor very uneasily and renders problematic whether this is a work of imagination or the chronicling of lived experience. In *4:48 Psychosis*, it is difficult to see much distance between the authorial voice and the material that is wrought into the play.

Greig (2001) says:

> '*4:48 Psychosis* sees the ultimate narrowing of Kane's focus in her work. The struggle of the self to remain intact has moved from civil war, into the family, into the couple, into the individual and finally into the theatre of psychosis: the mind itself. "And my mind is the subject of these bewildered fragments," the play's voice states. Yet, perhaps it is as well to be cautious here. Whose mind? The mind of the speaker of the words in the theatre, definitely, but does that directly mean the mind of the author?'
>
> (p. xvi)

4:48 Psychosis is not just about despair, it is also about guilt, psychotic guilt that is not driven by actual misdemeanours but by delusion. This is outlandish, fantastical guilt:

> I gassed the Jews, I killed the Kurds, I bombed the Arabs, I fucked small children while they begged for mercy, the killing fields are mine, everyone left the party because of me...
>
> (Kane, 2001: p. 227)

The play also describes visual and auditory hallucinations:

> I'm seeing things
> I'm hearing things
> I don't know who I am.
>
> (Kane, 2001: p. 225)

It is in the combative, often ironic interplay with doctors that the play moves away from the interior world to the carefully observed rituals, the culture of medicine. This approach towards the peculiarities of medicine that combines irony and comedy is not limited to Sarah Kane. Plautus in *The Brothers Menaechmus* utilised the same approach to good effect, the difference being that Plautus' play is a comedy and the treatment of doctors is part of the overall tone whereas Sarah Kane's play is bleak and dark. The treatment of doctors in her case has a comic effect but nevertheless it hardly relieves the undertow of anxiety and foreboding:

> Dr This and Dr That and Dr Whatsit who's just passing and thought he'd pop in to take the piss as well. Burning in hot tunnel of dismay, my humiliation complete as I shake without reason and stumble over words and have nothing to say about my "illness" which anyway amounts only to knowing that there's no point in anything because I'm going to die. And I am deadlocked by that smooth psychiatric voice of reason which tells me there is an objective reality in which my body and mind are one. But I am not here and never have been. Dr This writes it down and Dr That attempts a sympathetic murmur. Watching me, judging me, smelling the crippling failure oozing from my skin, my desperation clawing and all-consuming panic drenching me as I gape in horror at the world and wonder why everyone is smiling and looking at me with secret knowledge of my aching shame.

> (Kane, 2001: p. 209)

The ironic, light tone of the opening line – 'Dr This and Dr That' – gives the impression of a turning outwards but quite quickly follows a turning back inwards in the fashion of depressive narcissism where everything in the world relates back to the self. The perspective is of shame, guilt and deep-seated disgust with the self.

The monologue continues:

> Inscrutable doctors, sensible doctors, way-out doctors, you'd think were fucking patients if you weren't shown proof otherwise, ask the same questions, put words in my mouth, offer chemical cures for congenital anguish and cover each other's arses until I want to scream for you, the only doctor who ever touched me voluntarily, who looked me in the eye, who laughed at my gallows humour spoken in the voice from the newly-dug grave, who took the piss when I shaved my head, who lied, and said it was nice to see me. Who lied. And said it was nice to see me. I trusted you, I loved you, and it's not losing you that hurts me, but your bare-faced fucking falsehoods that masquerade as medical notes.

> (Kane, 2001: pp. 209–210)

The ambivalent attitude towards doctors and also towards the conceptualisation of mental anguish as chemical in origin, the scepticism about the treatment on offer, and the desire for a personal relationship that is thwarted and obstructed by the strictures of the regimen in hospital, these are reflected through a sensibility corroded by despair and despondency. *4:48 Psychosis* is ultimately about melancholic psychosis. It is a dramatic treatise on the inner, unseen and uncharted territory of anguish. Its power derives from the intensity of morbid feeling. It is unremitting in the exposure of what tortures the interior life and all this effected merely with words that emerge without any obviously coherent underpinning narrative. Madness is not given meaning nor is it made understandable in context. The abyss of despair is just that, an abyss that is inescapable and that is sordid and terrifying. The stage in *4:48 Psychosis* is the deranged mind on display and what we see is neither comforting, nor pleasing. When at the end the text reads, 'It is myself I have never met, whose face is pasted on the underside of my mind' (Kane, 2001: p. 245), we want to retort, 'it is not your face, not your identity that is pasted on the underside of your mind'. However, the tragedy is that in real life, the doctors were saying that all along, yet it was not a reassuring response and it certainly did not alleviate anguish and did not avert the fatal end in suicide for Sarah Kane herself, as it did not for the voice in her play.

References

Bentley, E. (1952) Introduction. In *Naked Masks: Five Plays* (L. Pirandello). EP Dutton.

Borges, J. L. (1964) *Labyrinths: Selected Stories and Other Writings*. Penguin Books.

Esslin, M. (2001) *The Theatre of the Absurd*. Methuen Drama.

Greig, D. (2001) Introduction. In *Complete Plays* (S. Kane). Methuen Drama.

Ionesco, E. (2000) *Rhinoceros, The Chairs, The Lesson*. Penguin Books.

Kane, S. (2001) *Complete Plays*. Methuen Drama.

Norton, D. F. & Norton, M. J. (eds) (2000) *David Hume: A Treatise of Human Nature Being an Attempt to Introduce the Experimental Method of Reasoning into Moral Subjects (Oxford Philosophical Texts)*. Oxford University Press.

Pinter, H. (1991) *Plays 1*. Faber and Faber.

Pinter, H. (1993) *Plays 4*. Faber and Faber.

Pirandello, L. (1988) *Collected Plays. Volume 2*. John Calder Publications.

Prince, M. (1905) *The Dissociation of a Personality: The Hunt for the Real Miss Beauchamp*. Oxford University Press.

Index

Compiled by Linda English

Plays and books are found under the author's name